The Hyper(in)visible Fat Woman

The Hyper(in)visible Fat Woman
Weight and Gender Discourse in Contemporary Society

Jeannine A. Gailey

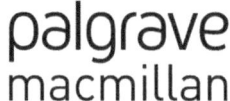

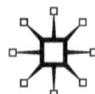

THE HYPER(IN)VISIBLE FAT WOMAN
Copyright © Jeannine A. Gailey 2014.

Softcover reprint of the hardcover 1st edition 2014 978-1-137-40716-0

All rights reserved.

First published in 2014 by PALGRAVE MACMILLAN® in the United States—a division of St. Martin's Press LLC, 175 Fifth Avenue, New York, NY 10010.

Where this book is distributed in the UK, Europe and the rest of the world, this is by Palgrave Macmillan, a division of Macmillan Publishers Limited, registered in England, company number 785998, of Houndmills, Basingstoke, Hampshire RG21 6XS.

Palgrave Macmillan is the global academic imprint of the above companies and has companies and representatives throughout the world.

Palgrave® and Macmillan® are registered trademarks in the United States, the United Kingdom, Europe and other countries.

ISBN 978-1-349-48810-0   ISBN 978-1-137-40717-7 (eBook)
DOI 10.1057/9781137407177

Library of Congress Cataloging-in-Publication Data

Gailey, Jeannine A., 1976–
  The hyper(in)visible fat woman : weight and gender discourse in contemporary society / Jeannine A. Gailey.
    pages cm
  Includes bibliographical references and index.

  1. Obesity in women—Social aspects—North America. 2. Body image in women—North America. 3. Discrimination against overweight persons—North America. I. Title.

RC552.O25.G35 2014
362.1963'980082—dc23   2014022208

A catalogue record of the book is available from the British Library.

Design by Scribe Inc.

First edition: November 2014

10 9 8 7 6 5 4 3 2 1

For Blake

Contents

Acknowledgments	ix
1 Hyper(in)visibility and the *Paradox* of Fat	1
2 Fighting the Fat Self	31
3 Fixing the Fat Body	57
4 Fit and Fat	83
5 Ample Sex	111
6 Embracing Fat Pride	137
7 Shifting the Focus	161
Appendix: Notes on Methodology	173
Notes	183
References	189
Index	203

Acknowledgments

This book would not have been possible without the generous support, guidance, and assistance of numerous people. First, thank you so much to each and every woman who took the time to talk with me and share your story. I am humbled by your generosity and trust. I am also incredibly grateful for the support I received from Texas Christian University and, more specifically, the Department of Sociology and Anthropology, the Institute on Women and Gender, the AddRan College of Liberal Arts, and the TCU Women's Studies Program for the generous financial support that made this research possible. There are several people within each of these departments and colleges who deserve mention: Morri Wong, Joanne Green, Andrew Schoolmaster, and Bonnie Melhart—thank you so much to each of you for all your encouragement and support throughout this project.

Several of my closest friends and colleagues not only supported and encouraged me throughout the research and writing process but also graciously gave their time to read and comment on various chapters, grant proposals, and ideas throughout this research process. Thank you so much Carol Thompson, Bob Young, Jeff Ferrell, Mike Katovich, Ariane Prohaska, Claudia Camp, Michaela Nowell, and Hathaway Roche. You have all greatly influenced my ideas and, in a variety of countless ways, helped me complete this book.

Moreover, I'm so grateful for my wonderful friends, family, and colleagues' unyielding support, encouragement, intellectual insight, and engaging conversations about this research over coffee and, occasionally, cocktails. Thank you so much Shannon Booth, Karen Lang-Ferrell, Jana Jackson Lloyd, Lisa Vanderlinden, Kika and Steve Sloan, Jean Giles-Sims, David Gunn, Tracie Harris, Sarah Hine, Shawn Keane, Pam Carlisle, Kerri, Jim, and Ben Mauro, Abby Baker, Claire Carroll, Matt Lee, Penny Owens, Claudia Schoenstein, Rita Logero, Robin Powell, Sharon Gailey, my mother, Linda, grandmother Thelma, and my much-missed father, George.

I'm also incredibly grateful that during this journey I had a fabulous writing partner, Lauren Jade Martin. Thank you for reading the chapters so closely and providing helpful commentary. I'm thrilled that you also received a book contract and am looking forward to seeing it in print.

Writing this book would not have been as fulfilling or intellectually stimulating had it not been for my wonderful partner, Blake Hestir. Blake has taken on this project like it was his own. He not only read each chapter multiple times and listened to me practice the talks I gave while writing the book but also provided extremely beneficial criticism and pushed me intellectually. I'm so grateful for his willingness to partake in the near-constant conversation about this research, all the news articles he sent me related to the topic, suggestions for the cover design, and feedback. In fact, Blake has been so incredibly enthusiastic about this project that he frequently would tell anyone who would listen about this research and how important he thinks it is. Thank you so much, Blake.

Finally, thank you Lani Oshima and Mara Berkoff at Palgrave Macmillan. You have been a wonderful editorial team and have been tremendously helpful and enthusiastic throughout the whole process.

Chapter 1

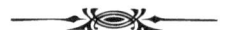

Hyper(in)visibility and the *Paradox* of Fat

Jennifer[1] is a 34-year-old woman from the upper Midwest in the United States. She is 5'2" and wears a size 22. She is unsure of her exact weight but guesses that she is around 230 pounds. Jennifer is considered "obese" by medical standards and has been so for most of her life. She was "average" size until she was eight years old but began gaining weight shortly thereafter. Her mother would often question how much she ate and began to restrict her food intake. Jennifer explained that she and her siblings would eat as much junk food as they could when their parents were away for the evening. She stated that this was probably a precursor to overeating, which she tends to do when she restricts her food intake or is upset or stressed. Recently she decided that she had to eat more healthfully and she eliminated processed foods and soda but reported that she always keeps sweets around because she is less likely to overindulge if they are available. She no longer diets because restriction, at least in her case, leads to overeating or bingeing.

Jennifer feels pretty good about herself on most days. She eats "intuitively" and stays active. She walks two miles each way to work every day, sometimes in freezing temperatures. She is in a positive, loving relationship, is highly educated and employed, and has an overall positive outlook on life. Jennifer is a successful, thirtysomething woman who, by most standards, is healthy. She does not have high cholesterol, diabetes, or high blood pressure. In many respects, Jennifer is the antithesis of what we think of when we think about an "obese" woman in contemporary society. Her story, it turns out, is not that unique.

Many of the women who are featured in this book have stopped dieting. They take care of their bodies and in myriad ways defy the stereotypes that many hold about "fat"[2] women. Some are reportedly not healthy (which may or may not be attributed to their weight); some are extraordinarily disappointed in their appearance; a number have had weight-loss surgery such as lap band or gastric bypass; and a few lead troubled lives for various reasons, not merely including the difficulties associated with being an "obese" woman in a fatphobic society. These women come from a range of backgrounds and places. Some have PhDs or law degrees. Others dropped out of high school. Some are from affluent backgrounds. Others are or were at one point impoverished.

But the one thing they all have in common is the stigma of being labeled "obese." In fact, most would be considered "super obese" or "obese class III" by medical standards, although they sometimes refer to themselves as "supersized" (see Appendix for more on the participants and methodology).

The heightened attention directed toward *obesity* by the media, politicians, the medical establishment, and the general public highlights the fact that the body, especially the fat body, is a site of significant social contest (cf. Pitts 2003). Fat is often discussed in hyperbolic terms of "fighting fat," "battling fat," or the "catastrophic effects of fat." One does not have to look very far to find what seems to be an endless stream of news articles, blogs, and opinion editorials about the "obesity epidemic" and the alleged threat it poses to our nation in terms of national security and health. For example, my online search of "news" and "fighting fat" returned 36,000 hits, "battling fat" yielded fewer at 5,700, and "catastrophic effects of fat" under "news" revealed 1,620 articles (November 28, 2012).

Social control over bodies is nothing new, especially women's bodies. In the nineteenth century, women wore corsets because those with small waists were granted higher social status and seen as more fertile, beautiful, and embodying true womanhood. Corsets frequently caused mobility and dressing problems, as well as broken ribs, punctured lungs, reproductive problems, and sometimes death. Today the most coveted womanly form is thin and toned, and similar to having a small waist, thinness confers social status and privilege. Many women go to extreme lengths to achieve this "ideal form," and sometimes the results are just as harmful as corseting.

The concern in the United States over the *obesity epidemic* has become one of the most popular social problems among politicians, the medical establishment, media outlets, and academics over the last decade. However, little research has been conducted from the perspective of fat persons in North America. The media and medical establishment argue that the attention serves as education about the dangers of fat and as motivation for weight loss, whereas Fat Studies scholars argue it leads to marginalization. Some research has indicated that size discrimination leads to a deterioration in health (Amy et al. 2006), lower academic achievement (Crosnoe 2007), lower wages (Averett and Korenman 1996), inadequate treatment by health-care professionals (Rothblum et al. 1990; Teachman and Brownell 2001; Young and Powell 1985), and an increase in disordered eating (Darby et al. 2009, 2007). Popular anecdotes for *obesity* prevention or reduction emphasize eating fewer calories and increasing activity. Yet there is evidence to indicate that this oversimplifies a rather complicated process that involves numerous social factors and biological differences (Ernsberger 2009).

Before I move on, I want to note why I am using the word *fat* and why I place quotes around the words "obesity," "overweight," and "obesity epidemic." I use the word *fat* not in a pejorative sense but as an adjective like those involved in field of Fat Studies (sometimes also known as Critical Weight Studies) and in the spirit of size acceptance. Fat Studies scholars argue that *obesity* is a highly contentious word that denotes a medical condition and problematizes human diversity. In these circles, *fat* is the preferred adjective because it does not denote a medical condition or suggest that there is an ideal weight, such as *overweight*. As Marilyn Wann (2009, xiii) states, "Medicalization of weight fuels anti-fat prejudice and discrimination in all areas of society." The supposition is that fat is not only an individual choice but also an irresponsible choice that must be cured to protect society.

In addition, calling *obesity* an epidemic has serious ramifications, as Samantha Murray (2008) points out in her book *The Fat Female*

Body. If a community is dealing with an epidemic, it is expected and understood that members of that community will do everything in their power to prevent the spread of the disease. It becomes a public duty, as well as a personal responsibility. However, "obesity" is not a communicable disease. In *Killer Fat* (2012), Natalie Boero explains that the term *epidemic* is increasingly used for diseases and other social phenomena that are not contagious and sometimes not even diseases. Boero argues that "obesity"—like the "teen pregnancy epidemic" or the "school violence epidemic"—is a "postmodern epidemic" because the term no longer implies a communicable disease. A postmodern epidemic is a human experience that is defined and treated as a medical condition but that is not inherently a medical condition (Boero 2012, 4).

I also use *large*, *plus size*, and *person of size* interchangeably with *fat* because not everyone I talked with was comfortable with the word *fat*. Many of the women referred to themselves as fat, even if they were not involved in size acceptance, but some of the women did not like the word *fat* and did not refer to themselves as fat, so when I refer to those specific women, I try to respect their choice in language.

In this book, I seek to answer the following questions: How do women of size negotiate a cultural landscape that is increasingly antifat? What impact does the "war on obesity" have on the way fat women are positioned in society? What are women's perspectives about their size, health, and body image? And how does that impact their sexuality and identity?

I begin with my motivation for beginning this project. In 2004, I read an article by Sarah Fenske in the Cleveland *Scene* magazine, "Big Game Hunters. Men Who Chase Chubbies for Sport and Pleasure: They Call It Hogging." The article focused on several men who used, and sometimes abused, large women for their own sexual gratification and as a form of entertainment. I was horrified at the way the men discussed the women as less than human—it was extreme objectification. Their actions were deplorable. I had never heard of hogging, but interestingly many of my male friends had.

A colleague and I designed a study to better understand the social forces that lead some men to act in such a way. We conducted 13 interviews with undergraduate, heterosexual men, because Fenske indicated that we should target that population. We found that 11 of the 13 knew about the practice and identified it by name, without us using the term *hogging*, and knew people who did it. In addition, all 13 thought it was funny (I discuss these findings in further detail in Chapter 5). Subsequent to sharing our findings (see Gailey and Prohaska 2006; Prohaska and Gailey 2010), we were frequently asked what the women say about it. This struck me as a good question, but we had not interviewed women, nor were we sure how to go about recruiting women for such a study.

Several years later, I discovered the National Association to Advance Fat Acceptance (NAAFA) through the work of Debra Gimlin (2002). Gimlin interviewed women involved in NAAFA about how they manage the stigma of fat. Relationships and meeting men was part of the conversation, although not the emphasis of her study. Many of the women were reportedly leery of the men they met at NAAFA functions because many of the men were fat admirers (Goode and Preissler 1984) or fat fetishists. A "fat admirer" is a man who prefers large women, although many are in the closet because of the stigma associated with fat.

Following this discovery, I read as much as I could about NAAFA and the size acceptance movement in general. In phase one of the present study, I recruited interviewees through the numerous size acceptance listservs, blogs, and social networking groups. For phase two, I expanded my recruiting efforts to include women not involved in size acceptance or who were likely unaware of the movement by posting invitations on my personal Facebook page and asking friends to share it, contacting bariatric surgery groups, and posting on numerous Yahoo! groups that were formed around "obesity" and weight loss. The total sample consisted of 74 women of size. The in-depth interviews were loosely structured and focused on the women's dieting and weight-loss histories, sexual and relationship histories, health, and identity politics (see Appendix for a detailed discussion of my methodology).

I should also mention that I am not a woman of size. I am petite and by most people's standards I would be considered thin or "average size" (5'2" and 115 pounds). I have never been fat or even "overweight," but like most people my weight has fluctuated somewhat over the years. Even though I have never been medically considered "overweight" or "obese," I have had other women call me fat in an attempt to hurt my feelings. But I cannot and do not deny the privilege I have experienced as a result of being "average sized," and I have never been discriminated against for my body size.

However, I have personally struggled with accepting my body, despite having never been "overweight." I went through puberty before most of my peers and have been roughly the same size since seventh grade. Physically developing so quickly made me extremely self-conscious, and I always felt larger than I actually am. I have engaged in numerous diets, including severely restricting my caloric intake and overexercising. I still exercise, but I no longer diet or exercise to burn off what I ate. In fact, discovering the size acceptance movement has helped me feel better about my body and become even more critical of media images of women and the messages propagated about dieting, weight loss, and the harms of fat.

I argue that this book is an important contribution because people of size have been the subject of a tremendous amount of critical attention in the media, medical profession, and by politicians, due to the alleged harms of "obesity" and the "obesity epidemic." Women tend to be disproportionately impacted by the "war on obesity" partly because women are expected to be beautiful, and fat is typically not considered beautiful. This book is centered on 74 fat women's experiences, respectfully bringing their voices to the forefront as they straddle a seemingly paradoxical social position that I term *hyper(in)visibility*.

The *Paradox* of Fat and the Spectrum of Visibility

In *Missing Bodies: The Politics of Visibility*, Casper and Moore (2009) use a comparative method to examine the politics surrounding bodily exposure and erasure. They argue that the dimensions of visibility depend on which category the body fits into. For example, when contrasting "innocent" and "heroic" bodies, Casper and Moore (2009, 181) equate the former as having limited exposure and the latter as experiencing surplus exposure.

Casper and Moore (2009, 15) propose a multidimensional method for analyzing missing bodies that they call the *ocular ethic*. The ocular ethic involves focusing, which is a close inspection of marginalized bodies with the tools of magnification, such as ethnography, to increase the attention on bodies that have been concealed. Bodies move in and out of visible and invisible spheres of perception, to such an extent that "the ocular ethic represents the responsibility that comes with seeing or perceiving bodies *and* identifying and recovering those bodies that are unseen or less exposed to the public eye" (Casper and Moore 2009, 186, emphasis in original). Their thesis not only remains provocative but also serves as a practical guide for me to navigate the spectrum of visibility, especially regarding fat bodies.

We learn in early childhood to observe others' bodies for social clues about their position in the social hierarchy (Casper and Moore 2009). Butler (1990) asserts that the materialization of bodies is essential to the creation of social and political life. Discourses and practices rely on the actions, interactions, and positioning of bodies. Some bodies are highly public, visually inspected, and made into a spectacle, while others are subject to discrimination or erasure because of societal stratification along the lines of class, race, ethnicity, gender, sexuality, age, ability, and so on (Casper and Moore 2009, 9). Fat presents an *apparent* paradox because it is visible and dissected publicly; in this respect, it is *hypervisible*. Fat is also marginalized and erased; in this respect, it is *hyperinvisible*.

Contemporary Western societies relegate fat women to a hyper(in)visible space, a phenomenon that occurs explicitly within institutions (e.g., hidden from view in corporate endeavors that show off thin women) and implicitly in our interpersonal and imagined worlds (through shunning or typecasting particular body types in everyday life and media). Moreover, the spectrum (see Figure 1.1) from hypervisible to hyperinvisible remains robust, intense, and deeply ingrained in our ceremonial social life. To be hyper(in)visible means that a person is sometimes paid exceptional attention and is sometimes exceptionally overlooked, and it can happen simultaneously. Fat women are hyperinvisible in that their needs, desires, and lives are grossly overlooked, yet at the same time they are hypervisible because their bodies literally take up

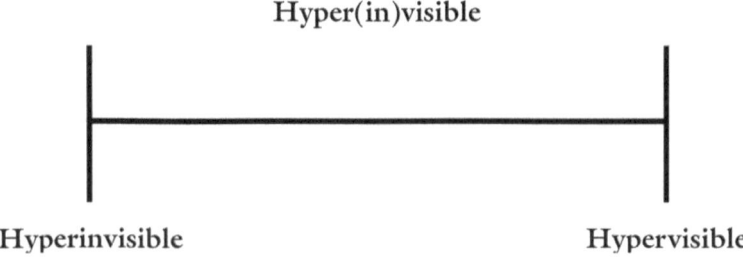

Figure 1.1 Spectrum of visibility

more physical space than other bodies and they are the target of a disproportionate amount of critical judgment.

In what follows, I discuss the spectrum of visibility and how others have conceptualized (in)visibility. I then turn to an explanation of the phenomenon of hyper(in)visibility. I argue that the prefix *hyper* is necessary to achieve the focus—the ocular ethic—needed to analyze marginalized bodies, groups, or ways of life. We are all visible and invisible at times (as I demonstrate in the following section), but one's situation becomes "hyper" when (in)visibility becomes socially oppressive.

The Spectrum of Visibility

Through appearance alone, embodied actors communicate our situated identities, including our present, past, and future existence as social beings that occupy various social places. Body size is similar to other nondiscursive appearances (race or ethnicity, sex, and gender) in that it is noticeable prior to any word utterances. Moreover, based on how these non-discursive social markers intersect, assumptions are made about that person.

For instance, a woman shopping at a moderately priced retail clothing store attracts immediate attention and evaluation within that context as merely embodied, independent of content and substance of speech. However, a thin white woman will likely be offered assistance more quickly than a thin Latina woman. This discrepancy in attention involves stereotypes associated with race and ethnicity. Sales clerks may incorrectly assume that the white woman can afford to purchase more than the Latina woman. But both of these women are appropriately gender identified—meaning their sex and gender identity correspond—and they are both thin (both privileged statuses). What would happen if one of the women were fat? Jennings (2010) asked a similar question. Using participant observation, she examined the treatment of fat customers and clothing option availability for plus-size women in various types of popular women's clothing stores. Jennings, a self-described fat white woman, details how sales clerks ignored her with systematic regularity. In contrast, sales clerks greeted, helped, and catered to "appropriately embodied" (thinner) customers. Jennings's fat body marked her as "out of place" in these retail stores. This singular experience of (in)visibility indicates the tremendous impact the size of our body has on the way we are treated in society and the privileges we are granted.

Visibility is intimately related to acknowledgment or recognition (Brighenti 2007). To be seen by a *significant other* means that we exist; in Mead's ([1934] 1967) terms, the significant other "tests" and "testifies" our existence by looking at us. Visibility has to do with subjectification and objectification—with the ontoepistemological (being and knowing) structure of objects and subjects (Brighenti 2007). In essence, one of the ways we come to know who we are occurs as we examine and acknowledge how others see us through the societally constructed prism that identifies the "normal." We in turn come to know ourselves as both a subject (idiosyncratic awareness of self) and an object (awareness of self from another's perspective). We know where we "belong" in society based on our estimation of how others locate and view us in social and societal terms (Stone 1962, 87–88). The "normal" body is socially recognized as evidenced by the smiles or nods of passing strangers, the fact that people will move out one's way when navigating through a crowded space, and through being waited on or helped when in a restaurant or store. Normalcy is regarded as being able-bodied, having light skin, having sex and gender congruity, and being thin or "average-sized," heterosexual, and middle-class.

There is a complex relationship between power and visibility, as Foucault and others have noted. But Foucault (1977) reminds us that visibility is deceptive. In some instances, being seen signifies respect as discussed before, but when being seen results in stares of disapproval, the act of being seen is *Othering*. Foucault discusses visibility in terms of power and discipline when he appropriates Bentham's panopticon to illustrate how constant visibility—being under surveillance—creates inequities and a mechanism of punishment. Bentham designed the panopticon to be a circular prison where the guards occupy a central watchtower from which they could monitor prisoner behavior while remaining invisible to the prisoners. Eventually, the prisoners, not knowing when they were or were not being watched, would police themselves, or in Foucault's terms, become "docile bodies" (Foucault 1977, 202). When applied to contemporary society, Foucault writes extensively about the regulating and normalizing gaze, which happens when people are under, or believe they are under, constant surveillance. People discipline themselves and police their behaviors because anyone could be watching. As Tischner (2013, 45) states, "Permanent visibility goes together with increasing individualization within a disciplinary system. While power itself becomes invisible . . . those subjected to the power become more and more visible." All bodies are subject to surveillance, but some bodies are watched more closely while other bodies disappear or seemingly vanish.

To be visible or seen is a form of acknowledgment—that one exists or matters—but at other times it means one is different and is subject to inspection or scrutiny. Queer persons, fat persons, persons of color, and bodies of persons with physical differences, such as those with missing limbs, scars, or those who engage in extreme body modification all experience visibility, but frequently in a socially oppressive way. However, as visible as they appear and feel, they also experience invisibility in numerous social contexts, to the extent that they become hyper(in)visible. They often notice disapproving stares and experience an intense "onstage" feeling as if judged and ridiculed with every move.

Contrast this treatment with the way that white (or light-skinned), middle-class, gender-conforming, thin, and heterosexual people move their bodies through social spaces with ease and confidence such that the sight of them evokes positive responses. According to Dolezal (2010), "The normal body is the invisible body; it is a healthy body, untroubled by illness, discomfort, or disability, which is furthermore socialized and normalized to behave within the standards dictated by its sociocultural context and to display a neutral physical aspect through a meticulous self-regulation with regard to appearance and comportment within intersubjective encounters" (362–63).

Privileged bodies are invisible. Their every move is not analyzed. They are frequently given quite a bit of latitude regarding their behaviors. For instance, they might cut in line, speak loudly on their cell phone, or cough without covering their mouth with minimal social repercussions. In other words, privileged bodies are visible when the situation suits them. For example, recall the thin white woman who experiences immediate catering in clothing stores but also enjoys an invisible status when she moves through customs while traveling. Her experience and status allows her a welcomed social invisibility, in which the person has a "visually unobtrusive body" that passes "unnoticed within the milieu of anonymity that is the hallmark of social relations" (Garland-Thomson 2004, 8).

Marginalized or "visually obtrusive bodies" typically become visible at inopportune times. Authorities might target them, or their immediate presence can draw stares or looks of disgust when they ask to have their needs accommodated. While socially invisible, they remain symbolically crucial (Rajaram and Grundy-Warr 2004). As crucial symbolic figures—such as persons of color, queer persons, disabled persons, and fat persons—they experience, simultaneously, deprivation of recognition and surplus attention. As Goffman (1971) noted in other contexts, our taken-for-granted public life involves a socially artistic mix of observing others, appearing to ignore others, and acknowledging others intermittently, without obtrusive intensity. Our artistry includes the motivation to be acknowledged, but only in the right way. We seek recognition for things defined as good, but we avoid standing out or drawing negative attention (Dolezal 2010). We wish for definitions of our capabilities rather than observations of our (socially constructed) flaws and incapacities.

Zitzelsberger (2005), for instance, uses visibility and invisibility to explain the perceptions of women with disabilities or differences, specifically with regard to their gendered and embodied lives. Zitzelsberger's participants' physical disabilities or differences were visible, although some women's disabilities or differences could be invisible/hidden depending on the context. Similar to the present study, these terms encompass visual representations of individuals, as well as other ways that the women are perceived and experienced by others and themselves. (In)visibility represents a paradoxical situation where the women were simultaneously seen and ignored.

The Phenomenon of Hyper(in)visibility

Previous research has focused on (in)visibility but has not moved beyond the dialectical relationship between the invisible and the visible to discuss how bodies are viewed at the extreme. I argue that the spectrum of visibility must include the two extremes of hyperinvisibility and hypervisibility to fully account for the paradoxical position of marginalized bodies and persons. Marginalized bodies are not just seen or acknowledged; they are dissected and overtly made into a spectacle. Similarly, marginalized bodies are not simply invisible—that is, easily moving through social situations without too much attention or unwarranted inspection—but also erased and entirely dismissed, as Rochelle (35, African American) describes: "During my teenage years when I was not as heavy, people spoke to me in public, they were nice. You could get friendly conversation out of a cashier or a passerby. During my heaviest and my late 20s, it was like, I know I'm the biggest person in here yet nobody actually sees me. It's almost like being invisible; people look right through you. Cashiers don't even look you in your eyes when they speak to you. Now, at my heaviest, no; it's like dismissive; you're just dismissed before you even can make your presence known." Rochelle describes her experience as an invisible woman, or as I argue, a hyper(in)visible woman. She notes that she has witnessed firsthand the difference in the way people treated her when she was not as heavy and at her heaviest. Hyper(in)visibility is a mode of Othering. Rochelle is more than invisible because people do see her; "she is the biggest person in here," but they intentionally dismiss her. Therefore, she is simultaneously seen and ignored—she is hyper(in)visible.

Rochelle is not alone. In the 74 interviews I conducted for this book and the countless manuscripts I have read that were written by and about people of size, including the size activist conversations that I have been exposed to, the phenomenon of hyper(in)visibility is pervasive in the lives of fat women—but it has yet to be discussed specifically in terms of hyper(in)visibility.

Consider another example of how hyper(in)visibility manifests in the lives of the women I interviewed. I include two different excerpts from the same woman to show how she is in one instance hyperinvisible and in the next hypervisible. In the first, Evelyn (32, white) is shopping for a strapless bra:

> This was three years ago. I walked into a store and there was a lady and she was like, "Can we help you find anything?" I said, "Well, I'm looking for a strapless bra to go with my bridesmaid's dress." She kind of stopped and kind of glances over me and then turns to her coworker and says, "Oh, I don't think we have anything in her size." I'm just kind of like standing there open-mouthed like, "What?" I was just shocked that she actually said that and she wasn't even addressing me. It was like I wasn't even there. She was talking to her coworker.

I should point out that Evelyn is at the very low end of the "obesity category"—in fact, she is well below the average of the sample of women in this study, yet she still has experienced hyper(in)visibility. This narrative indicates her "social strangeness," as one not belonging in this store. The sales associate does not treat her as an actual customer when it is clear that she is buying something for herself. She talks to the other sales associate as if Evelyn is not present—Evelyn is hyperinvisible. In the second narrative, Evelyn is negotiating a ride at an outdoor festival:

> At an Oktoberfest festival a couple of years ago, my husband and I had gone on a particular carnival ride and we decided we wanted to go on the ride again so we hopped off, got back in line, we waited in line for like a half hour. We get up there. We go to sit in the very first, the front seats, and we were trying to pull the safety harness down, but the hydraulics hadn't kicked in yet so it wasn't locking into place. The attendant that was there in broken English he was like, "You're too fat." I'm looking at him like, "What?" He's like, "You're too big." I said, "Are you telling me that I'm too fat to sit here?" He said, "Yes." Well, of course, the ride is like full at this point so this was happening in front of everybody else on the ride and so he's telling me that we need to move, that we need to change seats. Like the seats are going to be different sizes in another spot, you know?

Evelyn is hypervisible in that her body has now been put on display for everyone on the ride to see. She was publicly called out and shamed and then had to get up in front of everyone to move to a seat further back on the ride. She was not merely visible to others on the ride; she was made exceptionally visible—hypervisible. In both of these scenarios, Evelyn has been reduced to her body, and her body size has marked her as not belonging and resulted in her being treated without common courtesy or respect, which is how hyper(in)visibility plays out in the lives of fat women.

Throughout the remainder of the book, I focus on these 74 women's lives and provide further evidence for how hyper(in)visibility manifests in their lived experiences. However, before doing so, it is important to consider how the phenomenon of hyper(in)visibility works on both the structural and individual levels.

On the structural or societal level, hyper(in)visibility is primarily the result of messages projected by the media, medical establishment, and popular culture. The fat body is hypervisible in that it takes up a large amount of physical space, which is most evident on public transportation or in public venues, such as stadiums, classrooms, waiting rooms, medical facilities, and so forth. Our society is not built for large bodies partially because there is a pragmatic need to fit as many bodies as possible in places like classrooms, waiting rooms, airplanes, buses, or subways. Public space is frequently constructed based on profit rather than human comfort (Huff 2009).

Another reason large bodies are ignored is that historically they have been a minority. I spoke with several large women who are cancer survivors, and they talked about their frustration with the fact that they often could not fit on the medical equipment in hospitals and would sometimes have to travel several hundred miles to a location that could accommodate their bodies. Having to travel such great distances when they were sick made them feel like they were castaways, outsiders, aliens, or invisible, which on a structural level is how they are treated.

The medical establishment, politicians, and the media have pathologized "obesity" and labeled it a disease (Kwan and Graves 2013; Saguy 2013). Once framed in this manner, it is extraordinarily difficult to change the way the larger population views fat because it has been normalized as an illness as well as a moral failure (Saguy 2013). The emphasis on the "obesity epidemic" has also created a landscape where fat bodies are hypervisible (Boero 2012). Fat persons are routinely taunted, parodied, satirized, publicly condemned, and blatantly discriminated against (Andreyeva, Puhl, and Brownell 2008). Even fat persons with tremendous social capital feel the sting of hyper(in)visibility, such as New Jersey Governor Chris Christie, who had weight-loss surgery following harsh criticism about his weight. Some speculate that he had weight-loss surgery to improve his chances for a presidential run in 2016. In essence, he was too fat to appear presidential, so he had to surgically alter his body in order to lose enough weight to "look" like a president.

There is overwhelming evidence that antifat bias disproportionately impacts the lives of women (Fikkan and Rothblum 2012), yet many mainstream feminist scholars have not included fat women's bodies in their attempts to theorize the female body. On the other hand, anorexic bodies have been paid a tremendous amount of attention in the feminist literature on women's bodies.

Why do so many feminists study anorectics and so few study fat women? The answer is likely that fat has been framed as unhealthy and an individual problem, rather than a structural one (see also Saguy 2013). Anorexia is often considered to be the fault of society's preoccupation with thinness and patriarchy. By excluding or failing to focus on fat women's bodies, feminist scholars perpetuate the hyper(in)visibility of fat women's bodies and lives.

On an individual or experiential level, hyper(in)visibility takes place in interactions, through the internalization of fat hatred or embodiment of fat, and through the emphasis or de-emphasis of corporeal needs and desires. Symbolic interactionists Waskul and Vannini (2006) extend Cooley's (1902) concept of the "looking-glass self" by suggesting a "looking-glass body." Cooley's looking-glass self involves a process where one reflects and forms images of one's self from the imaginary perspective of others. The looking-glass body involves the idea that bodies are seen and the act of seeing is reflexive in the same way that Cooley identifies. When we look at others' bodies, we interpret what we observe and others imagine what we may be seeing and feeling—completing the reflection of the looking glass (Waskul and Vannini 2006, 5). The looking-glass body is not a direct reflection of others judgments; it is an imagined reflection, constructed from signals taken from others. In other words, we see our bodies from the perspective of others, or at least what we imagine others see.

This process of imagination and self-indication becomes all the more important when we think about the fat body. The fat body is heavily stigmatized and considered unattractive in Western society. Therefore, it is not surprising that the majority—if not all—of the women I interviewed at some point discussed feeling like others were judging them. They were aware of looks of disgust. They were sensitive to the inference that because their bodies are "so unsightly" they were completely ignored or erased from social situations.

The women whose voices are represented in this book indicated that they are often hyperinvisible when it comes to their health or actual dealings with health-care practitioners, in addition to frequently feeling invisible with sexual partners, family, friends, colleagues, and strangers. Throughout the interviews, women talked about growing up fat and struggling with kids at school teasing them or boys overlooking them. There were also cases where as children their pediatricians would react harshly to their weight but do so while talking to their parents as if they were not in the room—rendering them hyperinvisible. At work, discussions about weight, weight gain, and dieting occur frequently. Many of the women I interviewed talked about how they felt when their colleagues discussed these issues, especially because they are frequently the largest person in the room. Sometimes they became the focus of these conversations, albeit subtly. As one woman reported, someone would suggest, "We should start an office diet, don't you think?" and subsequently look at her, or they would act as if she (the interviewee) was not in the room—she is hyper(in)visible.

As a predicament and a performance, hyper(in)visibility symbolizes an accomplishment that emerges in social interactions. This symbolic accomplishment occurs when fat individuals, or formerly fat individuals who still see themselves as fat, engage in behaviors that perpetuate hyper(in)visibility. Just as those who "do gender" organize their activities to reflect or express gender and are disposed to see others' behaviors in a comparable fashion (West and

Zimmerman 1987, 127), "doing fat" means that fat persons also organize their actions to reflect or express being fat and see other fat persons similarly. For example, numerous women revealed that they thought they were "lucky" to have found men who are attracted to them or that they dated men who mistreated them because they did not think they would meet someone who would treat them with respect. They also talked about putting up with jobs where their employers took advantage of them by asking them to do things others would not. Jessica's narrative exemplifies how one does fat:

> I buried my sorrows alone in cartons of Ben and Jerry's—after all, isn't that what fat girls do?—and when at Mike's dorm I lost myself in 40 ounce bottles of malt liquor, and grain alcohol mixed with Hawaiian punch, and huge billowing hits from our father's handmade ceramic bong that Mike kept as an heirloom of sorts. I constantly ached for love and instead I would wake up in strange beds with strange men, faceless, nameless, all while I good-naturedly went along with Mike's jokes of "who wants to sleep with my sister?" After all, isn't that what fat girls do? I came to one night to find one of my brother's roommates thrusting into my mouth and when I burst into tears realizing that I didn't know how it had started he at least had the decency to stop. (Jessica, 35, white)

Jessica engaged in behaviors that she knows are stereotypical of fat women, but she said she did it because she felt isolated, unattractive, and Othered. As a young, fat woman, she felt out of place, unlovable, and abnormal. She said she did not respect herself because the cultural mandate is that fat people (especially fat women) are not respectable: They are gluttons, they overeat, and they cannot control their bodily urges the way that thin, disciplined women can. This pejorative comparison to thin women serves as an example of one mode of "doing fat"—that is, there are multiple ways of "doing fat." I discuss doing fat throughout the book, more specifically in Chapters 2 and 6.

Subsequently, fat women are regularly relegated and relegate themselves to the status of hyper(in)visible, a social location where they are sometimes passed over for job promotions, discriminated against in hiring and pay, have their ailments attributed to their size, and are ignored by the culture in a host of other ways.

They are marginalized and demonized. They are converted into the Other.

In sum, all bodies are sometimes visible or invisible, and as Star and Strauss (1999) argue, visibility and invisibility are "dialectically inseparable." I agree and contend that the concept of hyper(in)visibility demonstrates the dialectical relationship more clearly by showing how they work together, while accounting for bodies at the margins. The social position of fat women *seems* paradoxical because fat women suffer from both hypervisibility and hyperinvisibility, sometimes simultaneously. But while apparently paradoxical in the abstract, it also looms as a concrete fact about fat women's predicament in society. The reason that they are both is because of the extraordinary amount of attention their bodies are given in society through the "obesity epidemic" and stereotypes about fat people.

I close this conceptual discussion by sharing a quote from a woman who is a member of a size acceptance listserv, because she reports an experience that illustrates and symbolizes fat women's seemingly paradoxical position on the spectrum of visibility: "I had my TV on this morning . . . and all of a sudden the morning news anchor is almost screaming out the 'alarming news' that 'OBESE' WOMEN HAVE AN INCREASED RISK OF DEATH FROM BREAST CANCER!!! Good God. It really completely changed my mood from that of a peaceful and calm summer Monday morning to the grouchy thought that, 'Even if I live to be 110 my cause of death is going to be listed as "obesity" and I will be blamed for causing my own death by being fat.'" Her frustration with the way the media discussed and framed "obesity" exemplifies how fat women are positioned on the spectrum of visibility. The news sensationalized the story about "obesity" and breast cancer. "Obesity" is subjectively hypervisible, at least in the manner she perceived and retold the story. She then closes the discussion post with the thought that because of the hypervisibility of "obesity," her life or death will likely be reduced to her fat. Her feelings, preferences, beliefs, hopes, and so forth are not just invisible; she suffers hyperinvisibility because she and her feelings, needs, and experiences are erased and reduced to her body size.

Brighenti (2007) and Tischner (2013) both point out that visibility is a social process that involves the complicated intersections of one's social location (i.e., race/ethnicity, sex, gender, body size). Fat bodies, at least in contemporary Western culture, confer a low status in the social hierarchy because of the tremendous stigma associated with fatness, as we saw earlier. The fat body is usually only visible at the margins of society, and this typically includes a pathologizing narrative where fat is unhealthy and caused by irresponsibility (Kent 2001; Saguy 2013). In a neoliberal context, fat persons have a duty to "police" their behaviors—to become "docile bodies" under the normalizing and regulating gaze (Foucault 1977). Visibility serves as a mode of discipline where each person in the society is expected to act according to the norms for the good of society (cf. Tischner 2013). Both ends of the spectrum are oppressive and disempowering, which is why I argue the prefix *hyper* is necessary to understand the predicament and phenomenon of hyper(in)visibility. Throughout the remainder of this book, I employ Casper and Moore's (2009) ocular ethic to magnify fat bodies so that social oppression of fat women becomes transparent and the paradox of hyper(in)visibility is no longer hidden.

"Obesity" and the "Obesity Epidemic"

Warnings about the dangers of "obesity" and suggestions for how to lose weight are ubiquitous on television, radio, billboards, and from our physicians and health-care providers. It is difficult to walk down a city street, drive on a highway, turn on the television or radio, or surf the Internet without some sort of advertisement for weight-loss products. Many advertisements purport that weight loss offers improvements to health and body image, with statements like, "Lose weight and look and feel great." The implication is not only that bodies with fat on them are unattractive but that fat people are unhealthy and do not feel good about themselves. Moreover, the medical establishment tends to reinforce the message that there is a causal relationship between weight and health. Some researchers have found that the relationship between weight and health is not so clear and have suggested more precise measures of *actual* health (see Chapter 4 for a more thorough discussion).

Television shows such as *The Biggest Loser* are widely popular, as was the 2012 HBO four-part documentary series *Weight of the Nation*. *The Biggest Loser* first aired in 2004 and is now broadcast in more than 90 countries. It has also become, according to the show's website, "a leading health and lifestyle brand," generating more than $300 million in spending at more than 25,000 major retailers.[3] Contestants on the show compete over who can lose the most weight through drastic diet changes and exercise with the assistance of a personal trainer. Some of the contestants have achieved the constructed ideal of weight loss combined with successful weight management. But others have come forward to point out that behind the scenes the show promotes unhealthy weight loss through questionable means.[4] In addition to allegedly promoting unrealistic weight loss, the show perpetuates the larger societal view that losing a significant amount of weight is achievable through hard work—as if fat and laziness are interrelated.

In the United States, and many other cultures, body size is assumed to be an individual choice and within one's control. Many attribute being fat to overeating, lack of exercise, making bad decisions regarding the kinds of food to eat, or some combination thereof. Again the message is clear: People are fat because they are lazy, ignorant, gluttonous, and irresponsible. In addition to discrediting fat persons' willpower and moral fortitude, our society also tends to blame fat persons for increasing health-care costs, and some have gone so far as to claim fat people are contributing to climate change and high unemployment rates. The *Weight of the Nation* website purports that "obesity in America has reached a catastrophic level. Almost every aspect of our lives is threatened. The first step toward ending the damage is learning how to fight back."[5] This is powerful rhetoric, and some are concerned that the "war on obesity" is actually a "war on fat people" (Puhl, Peterson, and Luedicke 2012; Wann 2009), which could further mistreatment and discrimination in society.

According to the Centers for Disease Control and Prevention (CDC) in 2010–11, more than one-third of US adults were "obese" (BMI 30 or greater). BMI, or body mass index, is measured by dividing one's weight by his or her square height. BMI is used to determine if a person is underweight (BMI less than 18.5), normal (BMI above 18.5 but below 25), overweight (BMI 25 to 29), or obese (BMI 30 or greater). And note that these categories are not static: In June 1998, 30 million people woke up "overweight" or "obese" without gaining a pound because the overweight category was lowered from 27 to 25 and "obese" was lowered from 32 to 30 (Squires 1998). Paul Campos (2004) in his book *The Obesity Myth* and J. Eric Oliver (2006) in his book *Fat Politics* discuss the close ties between the diet industry, pharmaceutical companies, and researchers with grants from institutions such as the NIH (National Institute of Health). In other words, the change in BMI categories were likely the result of pressure from the diet and pharmaceutical industry that have much to gain if millions of people are labeled "overweight" or "obese" (see also Boero 2012).

Moreover, BMI is problematic (Burgard 2009; Campos et al. 2006; Campos 2004) because it does not measure the actual percentage of body fat, nor does it take into account body type (e.g., apple or pear shape). For example, some athletes may have a higher BMI because of the large amount of muscle mass on their bodies. Another major concern is that BMI is used to establish a normative weight range for people from a variety of backgrounds and shapes.

Despite these problems, most health-care practitioners argue that it is still the best measure of adiposity. Paul Ernsberger, a biomedical researcher at Case Western Reserve, argues that overall body size is likely related to health, but body size is largely determined by genetics and environment and is not likely to change by the loss of body fat. In fact, "reducing fatness of the body is unlikely to produce lasting health benefits that are claimed by promoters of weight loss" (Ernsberger 2012, 11).

The CDC warns that we must keep track of "obesity" rates because "obesity" poses serious health risks. The health risks that are often purported to increase as weight increases include certain types of cancer, Type 2 diabetes, coronary heart disease, liver and gallbladder disease, sleep apnea, hypertension, high cholesterol, stroke, and fertility problems. The issue that seems to be the most widely discussed as of late is Type 2 diabetes. According to the CDC, nearly 26 million Americans have Type 2 diabetes, and most of these cases are preventable with weight loss and exercise. However, one additionally learns on the CDC website that Type 2 diabetes is also heritable and is more likely to be present in certain racial/ethnic groups, those over 45, and persons who are not active.

An increase in Type 2 diabetes could be related to food quality, considering that corn syrup and other sugars are used in the majority of processed foods (Goran, Ulijaszek, and Emily 2013), lack of exercise (the majority of Americans are inactive; Colberg et al. 2010), an ageing population (Kirkman et al. 2012), or the increase in racial and ethnic minority populations in the United States (Oldroyd, Banerjee, Heald, and Cruickshank 2005). While it might be possible for some to prevent Type 2 diabetes, it is pretty clear that this is not the case for everyone. One can speculate that the increase in diabetes in the United States is related to the complex interaction between social class, race/ethnicity, age, activity level, and food quality, availability, and affordability.

A recent study refutes the claims that weight gain causes diabetes and indicates that diabetes or prediabetes precedes weight gain (Rebelos et al. 2011). Moreover, some studies claim that health is best measured by fitness level, rather than body weight or BMI (Ortega et al. 2012), and several have shown that extreme thinness is associated with increased mortality and that moderate "obesity" is associated with lower mortality (Campos et al. 2006; Ernsberger and Haskew 1987; Garner and Wooley 1991; Jerant and Franks 2012). Others have indicated that the relationship between poor health outcomes among those labeled "obese" may be related more to histories of weight cycling, health consequences associated with discrimination and stigma, and the fact that many fat persons tend to avoid physicians and preventive care for fear that they will be chastised for their weight (Ernsberger 2009; Lyons 2009).

Many within the medical community claim that fat causes ill health. However, the problem with the medical establishment's position is that it tends to confuse causation with correlation and defines optimal health within a narrow weight range without sufficient empirical evidence to substantiate it. These misleading messages then spill over into popular culture, where they are further perpetuated as fact. For example, in *Weight of the Nation*, Episode 1, the lead physician from the Bogalusa study states, "The obesity that we're seeing is very damaging to the cardiovascular system" (approximate time in the show 10:20). Several minutes later during the discussion about diabetes, another physician states, "It's the obesity that's the central driving force for the insulin resistance." Both of these physicians are making causal claims that obesity causes heart disease and diabetes, neither of which has been proven empirically. Both the media and medicine have worked in concert to frame "obesity" itself as illness, pathology, laziness, and gluttony. Once labeled a disease[6] it is hard to change societal views because of the norms of the medical field and larger culture (cf. Saguy 2013).

Why do both the media and medical establishment overemphasize the relationship between weight and health? Clearly, there are plenty of fat people who are unhealthy, but they are not unhealthy *just* because they are fat. They are unhealthy because they have high blood pressure, diabetes, or any variety of other conditions that are sometimes correlated with fat but not clearly caused by fat. What is more, there are plenty of "obese" people who are no more and no less healthy than people who fall within the range of what the medical establishment considers a "normal" weight. Conversely, there are plenty of Americans who fall well within their "healthy" or "ideal" weight range, yet suffer from a variety of serious ailments, including diabetes, hypertension, and heart disease. My point of contention with the medical establishment is the claim that fat causes ill health or even the assumption that we can determine how healthy someone is by how much he or she weighs.

The problem with portrayals of fat in shows like *The Biggest Loser* or *Weight of the Nation* is that they reinforce stereotypes that associate fat and "obesity" with unattractiveness and lack of willpower, not to mention that they perpetuate the faulty causal claim that fat causes ill health. Fitness, health, and popular culture magazines, books, blogs, and websites tend to overstate the relationship between weight and health, too, in addition to featuring models whose bodies are airbrushed and sculpted using computer software. We are led to believe that it is not only desirable but also possible to achieve a body that is remarkably thin and muscular, even though the models themselves do not actually look like the marketing copy.

The medical establishment, media, politicians, and political agencies, such as the CDC, work together to present a framework that fat causes ill health and people who fat are undisciplined, ignorant, or irresponsible. A recent Internet search with the key words *obesity* and *CDC* took me to a page on the CDC's website that promoted the HBO series *Weight of the Nation*. The *Weight of the Nation* website features physicians whose pictures are displayed to promote integrity to the films. When it comes to the concerns about "obesity" in the United States, it appears that there is a "Fat Industrial Complex" taking shape where medicine, government, entertainment, and political interests have all come together. One could speculate that the reason misinformation is perpetuated is because it takes the focus away from the real problems, such as food quality, the diet industry, stratification, and inequality. It is much easier to blame individuals than it is to change the structure of society.

"Obesity" is shrouded in what Goffman (1963) referred to as a discrediting attribute. While Goffman's work does not specifically focus on fat as a stigmatized identity, his concepts are useful for understanding fat stigma in the United States (Farrell 2011; Saguy and Ward 2011). Moreover, because fatness is a "discrediting attribute," many go to extreme measures to eliminate their fat. The multimillion-dollar diet industry provides plentiful evidence of the lengths to which people will go financially and physically to lose weight. This is because fat has been constructed into a physical stigma or an "abomination of the body"—one that is clearly visible. People cannot hide their fat. They literally wear their stigma on their bodies for everyone to see. Fat is the scarlet letter marking the fat woman's body. Fat is also a character stigma because our culture attributes many highly speculative and judgmental descriptions to fatness beyond the actual physical trait—fat persons are considered lazy, indulgent, out of control, or to be suffering from a psychological disturbance. Given the tremendous stigma associated with corpulence, it is not surprising that discrimination, mistreatment, and humiliation are common occurrences in the lives of people who are fat.

The women of size I talked with discussed the many assumptions people make about them because of their bodies. Almost every woman spoke about feeling like she had to prove that she was not lazy, dumb, or incompetent. Research on the discrimination of people of size has found that they are less likely to be hired, be promoted, earn more, get married, attend college, and receive adequate care from health-care practitioners (Ernsberger 2009; Rothblum et al. 1990; Teachman and Brownell 2001;

Young and Powell 1985) than their thin counterparts. This trend is exacerbated when we consider the lives of fat women (Fikkan and Rothblum 2012). The history and prevalence of fat hatred has been documented fairly well in the literature. However, few have focused on how persons overcome (if they even do) the internalization of fat hatred (I discuss this in further detail in Chapters 2 and 6). Goffman's (1963) work suggests that those who are stigmatized employ various forms of resistance. One key way that people cope with adversity is to connect with others who are similarly denigrated. The size acceptance movement, which formed in the late 1960s, has provided one such forum for resistance and community strength.

The Size Acceptance Movement

The size acceptance movement is a tapestry of organizations and individuals all over the world, but it started with the founding of NAAFA in 1969. William Fabrey founded NAAFA in part because he saw the discrimination his wife endured and how awful it made her feel about her body. In the early days of NAAFA, the organization focused on social aspects and was seen as a safe haven for fat women and their admirers. Dances and swim parties were common occurrences. In recent years, NAAFA has become more focused on the civil rights aspects of the movement. Activists, scholars, and members meet yearly at the annual convention and discuss everything from policy proposals to the best places to find clothing that can accommodate those at the heavier end of the weight spectrum. According to the NAAFA website, the mission of the organization is to "eliminate discrimination based on body size and provide fat people with the tools for self-empowerment through public education, advocacy, and support."[7]

The Fat Underground (FU), formed in California in the early 1970s, was the grassroots arm of the movement. Part of the reason FU formed was because they felt that NAAFA was not radical enough. They staged public demonstrations where they argued that the medical profession wanted to eradicate fat people, and according to Charlotte Cooper, a writer and fat activist, they were visionaries. They wrote the Fat Liberation Manifesto, which drew links between various forms of oppression and demanded equal treatment. The manifesto closed with the call: "Fat people of the world, unite! You have nothing to lose" (Freespirit and Aldebaran 2009, 342). The Fat Underground no longer exists as a group, but many of the living members are still active in the size acceptance movement.

Allen Steadham founded the International Size Acceptance Association in 1997, and while most of its branches are located in the United States, it does have some offices in other countries. The Internet, or "fat-o-sphere," also provides a whole host of size acceptance groups, forums, blogs, and social networking sites. Recent years have also seen the advent of a new academic discipline known as Fat Studies. *The Fat Studies Reader* was published in 2009, and in 2012 the inaugural issue of *Fat Studies: An Interdisciplinary Journal of Body Weight and Society* was published. Fat Studies scholars employ a critical eye by questioning claims that link fat to ill health and that keep fat people oppressed and feeling poorly about themselves. They ask questions about who benefits from the framing of "obesity" as an epidemic, and they seek to end discrimination and marginalization of fat people. The area of scholarship is growing, but it is not fully recognized, and it is still sometimes difficult to publish work that challenges the status quo in mainstream academic journals.

There are also BBW (Big Beautiful Women) groups all over the United States that host events such as pajama parties, breakfasts, potlucks, dances, and a variety of other events and outings. Some BBW events are specifically aimed at matching BBW and fat admirers (men who prefer fat women), but others are focused on creating networks of friends and hosting social events. About 15 of the women I interviewed had attended BBW events as a way to meet other people, sometimes for the purpose of dating, but frequently that was not the intention.

Not all size activism happens within organizations. There are several notable activists who have written books, speak publicly, and blog about discrimination, fatphobia, and misinformation presented in the media and academic literature on fat. Marilyn Wann's book *Fat!So?* was mentioned repeatedly by interviewees as a book that changed their lives. In addition, Charlotte Cooper's book *Fat and Proud* (1998) provides an excellent overview of the history of the fat acceptance movement, and activists Virgie Tovar and

Rebecca Weinstein have also recently published books that are popular and aimed at shifting the views about fat people, *Hot and Heavy: Fierce Fat Girls on Life, Love, and Fashion* (2012) and *Fat Sex* (2012), respectively.

An Overview of the Book

The remainder of the book consists of six chapters, including the conclusion. In Chapters 2 through 6, I focus specifically on how these 74 women discussed several aspects of their lives as they negotiate the phenomenon of hyper(in)visibility. In Chapter 2, I argue that societal fatphobia works to reinforce hyper(in)visibility on the experiential level through the internalization of fat hatred. The women's voices guide us through the daily trials and tribulations they encounter being fat. It impacts their view of self, others, their identity, and their actions. The phenomenon of hyper(in)visibility leads to (1) attempts to distance oneself from one's fat (it is not the real me or it is temporary) and (2) efforts to perpetuate "doing fat." However, a few of the women have begun to embody their fat (self) and shift the perspective about what it means to be a fat woman.

Chapter 3 focuses on three main issues: (1) how others have tried to contain participants' fat bodies; (2) how participants have attempted to expel their fat; and (3) those who have quit trying to "fix" their body. As they negotiate various diets and weight loss, and ultimately struggle with regaining weight, their bodies become both highly visible and invisible. Fat women are typically hypervisible when eating in public, shopping at the grocery store, or exercising at the gym. They are rendered hyperinvisible when they exhibit disordered eating behaviors for weight loss and as consumers of exercise clothing and accessories, which makes it even more challenging for them to engage in public exercise activities.

In Chapter 4, I argue that the neoliberal focus on health (especially the assumption that thinness signifies health) perpetuates the hyper(in)visibility of fat women. To demonstrate this process, the women's voices guide the reader through the complex notions of what constitutes health in their eyes and how they have been treated in the health-care system. The phenomenon of hyper(in)visibility is reinforced when physicians attribute any and all health ailments to participants' size while simultaneously rendering participants' knowledge of their own bodies and symptoms invisible. Hyper(in)visibility is further maintained when equipment, gowns, and medical screening devices cannot physically accommodate the bodies of larger persons. A substantial proportion of the women I interviewed discussed the Health at Every Size (HAES)® framework as an alternative to the hegemonic health paradigm. HAES® emphasizes physical fitness and healthful eating while ignoring how much one weighs.

Fat women tend to be viewed as either nonsexual or overly sexual, because they are typically viewed as simultaneously masculine and feminine. The bodily shame that most participants feel or have felt about their bodies is a predominant theme. The embodiment of shame contributes to the performance of hyper(in)visibility, where women of size position themselves as "Other" by sometimes engaging in stereotypical behaviors. In Chapter 5, the women's voices guide us through their dating and sexual histories and demonstrate how the phenomenon of hyper(in)visibility plays out in this aspect of their life. In addition, I highlight the various techniques these women used to transgress the way they see their bodies and subvert some of the negative messages.

In each of these chapters, I demonstrate that there are fat women who transgress bodily norms by accepting (or trying to accept) their body despite how incredibly challenging it is to be a fat woman in contemporary society. A sizable proportion of this sample either (1) accepts their body (or is in the process of acceptance) but does not identify with the size/fat acceptance movement or (2) embraces a fat identity through involvement (even minimal involvement) in the size/fat acceptance movement. In Chapter 6, I discuss the size acceptance movement and the politics of a fat identity, the embodiment of a fat identity, the resistance strategies employed by the women who challenge the dominant framework, and the ways in which activists "do fat" in order to upend the oppression of hyper(in)visibility. I also draw attention to some of the limitations of the movement and the difficulties women experience embodying a fat identity.

In the conclusion, I focus on the heuristic and academic importance of the concept of hyper(in)visibility for discussing marginalized bodies. The concept has broad application and illustrates how interactions and societal messages reinforce and perpetuate inequality. I asked each woman why she agreed to participate in the project, and nearly every woman explained that she hoped her story would help others. I discuss how I accomplished that goal, or at least tried, by using the women's standpoints to direct the writing of the book and the presentation of their stories. I offer modest suggestions for shifting the focus away from body weight to an emphasis on the appreciation of the diversity of human bodies, and I offer insights regarding how to subvert the hegemonic discourse.

Chapter 2

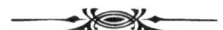

Fighting the Fat Self

As I discussed in the previous chapter, fat women are considered deviant and are stigmatized (Cahnman 1968; Cooper 2009; Farrell 2011; Puhl et al. 2012; Saguy and Ward 2011; Wann 2009; Schur 1984). Goffman (1963, 3–4) conceptualized stigma as a "deeply discrediting attribute" that classifies a person as dangerous or unacceptable based on three accounts: (1) a tribal stigma (i.e., race, nation, and religion that are transmitted through lineages), (2) an abomination of the body (i.e., various physical deformities), and/or (3) a blemish of individual character (i.e., weakness, dishonesty, mental disorders, etc.). For instance, fat persons are stereotyped as dumb, lazy, and irresponsible and are typically characterized as ugly, disgusting, and unkempt. For many, fat is so abhorred that even seeing or reading about fat people conjures feelings of disgust and anger, presumably because of the common perception that the fat person (woman) has "let herself go" or has "allowed herself" to become unkempt.

This stigmatized status reduces fat women to their bodies. As Moon and Sedgwick (2001) suggest, many people—upon seeing a fat woman—think that they know something about her, maybe even something that she does not know about herself. I frequently hear people say things such as, "Why is she wearing/doing/eating that? Doesn't she know how fat she is?" The common unspoken response is that we all *know* why she's fat. Our "collective knowledge" tells us that she is fat because she does not exercise, she overeats or eats fatty/sugary foods, or she does not take care of herself (Murray 2005). She is considered to be responsible or at fault for her size—she suffers the predicament of hyper(in)visibility.

Hyper(in)visibility works to oppress women by bringing a tremendous amount of attention to women (and others) who transgress bodily and aesthetic norms—by being fat—while simultaneously erasing or dismissing these women in social situations. Mistreatment and discrimination against fat persons is deeply embedded within the cultural ethos. Even racial or ethnic groups, such as African Americans and Latinos, that tend to celebrate larger women's bodies place limits on how large a woman can be before she is deemed unacceptable. However, research increasingly (DeAngelis 1997; Perez and Joiner 2003; Silber 1986) indicates that as Latinos and African Americans move into or above middle-class status, the preferred size of women's bodies decreases and begins to mirror that of the predominately Western European preference. Moreover, according to Beauboeuf-Lafontant (2003), the Black community respects large Black women, but their deviance—that is, their fat—is not necessarily loved. In other words, to be a large Black woman is symbolic of the strength that is expected of Black women but is not necessarily symbolic of beauty.

White women are not immune from the assumptions and expectations made about body size and social class. As Saguy (2013, 19) argues, "White women have more class and racial privilege to lose by being fat, whereas the prospects of women of color of all sizes are limited by racism." Typically the more money and wealth one has, the thinner they "ought" to be. In fact, body size (thinness) is a form of cultural capital and demonstrates "conspicuous leisure" (Veblen [1899] 1994). Veblen conceptualized conspicuous leisure as public displays of leisure time, such as playing golf or boating. Leisure is a privilege that the poor and working class do not typically have (see also Kwan and Graves 2013). Thinness demonstrates conspicuous leisure, because we typically associate thinness with exercise and "proper nutrition" (even though it is possible for someone to be unhealthy and thin). For most people, being thin requires time and monetary investment. Those in the lower socioeconomic strata do not typically have the luxury of disposable income or the time required to exercise and prepare meals from scratch. Moreover, since fat has been associated with the poor and persons of color, some have argued that the "war on obesity" is partly fueled by a desire to place symbolic distance between the affluent and those of lower socioeconomic status (Boero 2012; Saguy 2013).

Saguy and Ward (2011) conceptualize "fatphobia" as similar to homophobia, in that fat invokes tremendous hatred and fear. Fatphobia exists in contemporary society because thin bodies are prized and are considered medically, aesthetically, and morally desirable, while fat bodies are denigrated (54). Fat is so detested that "no one wants to be fat." In fact, many people adopt surprisingly radical means to eliminate (or attempt to eliminate) their fat, as I demonstrate in Chapter 3. This fear of "becoming"—in multiple senses of "becoming," such as actually gaining weight but also "becoming" as defining one's orientation toward others—or being fat, combined with the hatred and revulsion of fat, contributes to seeing oneself through the eyes of discriminating others. Many of the women I interviewed saw themselves in the predicament of the "less than" or the "inferior"—as beings deserving of mistreatment. In this regard, they were ugly and lazy humans positioned as the Other; in this way, they "became" fat.

In this chapter, I argue that societal fatphobia works to reinforce hyper(in)visibility on the experiential level through the internalization of fat hatred. The women's voices guide us through the daily trials and tribulations they encounter *being* fat. It impacts their view of self, others, their identity, and their actions. The phenomenon of hyper(in)visibility leads to (1) attempts to distance oneself from one's fat (i.e., fat is not the "real me" or it is merely temporary)[1] and (2) efforts to perpetuate "doing fat." However, a few of the women have begun to embrace their fat (selves) and shift the perspective about what it means to be a fat woman.[2]

Before moving forward, it is important to define what I mean by *self* and *identity*. The self includes—among other things—a system of ideas, attitudes, values, and commitments. The self is a person's total subjective environment; it is the unique or individual center of experience and significance (Jersild 1952, 4). George Herbert Mead ([1934] 1967), an American social theorist regarded as one of the founders of social psychology, argued that the self emerges out of the mind, the mind develops from social interaction, and patterned social interaction forms the basis of social structure. The mind is the thinking part of the self. It finds meaning for itself and others through language, where meaning is formed from symbols; the self is a social process.

An integral part of the self concerns reflexivity. Reflexivity, or self-awareness, refers to the ability of individual humans to place themselves perceptually as both objects and subjects. We get angry with, talk to, encourage, and congratulate ourselves much as we do one another. Our self becomes present to us as we act toward ourselves in the same manner that we act toward others. The ability to be reflective—to take oneself as an object—is the trait, according to Mead, that separates us from other animals (Gecas and Burke 1995; Mead [1934] 1967). "The organized community or social group which gives to the individual his unity of self may be called 'the generalized other.' The attitude of the generalized other is the attitude of the whole community" (Mead [1934] 1967, 164).

The self becomes a social entity, which emerges through the social process of adopting the attitudes and beliefs of an organized society or social group with which one is engaged.

Sheldon Stryker (1980) argues that the "self reflects society." He contends that the self is organized into multiple identities, each of which is tied to aspects of the social structure. One has an identity, an "internalized positional designation" (Stryker 1980, 60), for each of the different role relationships the person holds in society; in essence, we have multiple identities. In short, identity refers to the various meanings attached to the self, and it is considered to be the most public aspect of the self (Alexander and Wiley 1981).

There are multiple views of identity and identity theory in sociology (see Stryker 2000 for a review). I employ the view developed from Stryker and colleagues (Serpe and Stryker 1987; Stryker and Serpe 1982, 1994) that social structure influences one's identity and behavior. According to Stryker (1980), the numerous role identities that each person has are organized in a "salience hierarchy." A salient identity is one that is likely to be played out frequently across multiple situations and in numerous interactions. The salience of an identity is related to the degree of commitment one has to the identity, both qualitatively and quantitatively. For instance, if one has a great number of people with whom they interact in a particular identity and those ties are strong, then that identity is going to be more salient—in other words, the greater the commitment, the higher the identity is in the salience hierarchy (Stryker 1968, 1980).

The cultural condemnation and denigration of fat typically leads many fat persons to view their bodies as a temporary state to be overcome through diet, exercise, or some other weight-loss program.

They do not identify as fat and typically try to distance themselves from their fat. However, identity is an important component to social movements, which typically stress group identity in order to strengthen politically oppressed groups through (1) improving members' sense of confidence and (2) increasing the visibility of the oppression experienced by the group and its members. Therefore, fat women involved in the size acceptance movement may find it easier to *become* fat (i.e., embrace their body and identify as fat; Gailey 2012) than women who share the larger society's fatphobic views and stereotypical expectations of fat persons.

Remaining Hidden

Fat women, as a stigmatized group, are painfully aware of the fact that they are surreptitiously surveyed and monitored and simultaneously interactionally ignored, which enhances the salience of that identity and problematizes the negotiation (Goffman 1963; Kitsuse 1980). For instance, they can embrace the identity (become fat), attempt to neutralize the identity (fat is temporary), or symbolically distance their selves from the identity (I'm more than fat). However, the latter two options both involve hiding an aspect of one's self.

The metaphor of "being in the closet" is most commonly associated with someone who identifies as homosexual and "comes out of the closet" to denote his or her embodiment of a homosexual identity. Sedgwick (1993) states, "There *is* such a process as *coming out as a fat woman*" (230, emphasis in original; see also Saguy and Ward 2011). Both coming out as gay and coming out as fat are risky because both declarations, "I'm gay" or "I'm fat," come with years of hatred, discrimination, and Othering. When people who are gay stay in the closet, it is typically because they fear the social, and potentially physical, repercussions from their church, families, friends, colleagues, and so forth. In fact, some are quite successful at "passing as straight," and some may also be concerned that if they come out they will jeopardize the privilege they experience passing as heterosexual.

"Passing as thin" is not an option for someone who is fat.[3] So to come out as fat means that one is no longer ashamed of one's fat body. "They have come out to challenge conventional conceptions and judgments of their conduct, to question 'expert' assessments of their disabilities, 'handicaps' and devaluation of their capabilities, to reject the diagnosis of their various conditions and the attendant prescriptions for corrective treatment, and to publicly demand their rights to equal access to institutional resources" (Kitsuse 1980, 3). Coming out tells the world that regardless of what others might think of her, she has renegotiated her relationship with herself (body image and identity) and with others. Most of the women I spoke with have not come out as fat. In fact, the majority were actively trying to lose weight and were employing the social-psychological process of social distancing to separate their (true thin) self from that of "those fat people."

Samantha Murray (2005) outlines a few of the problems with coming out as fat and explains why the majority of fat people do not embrace a fat identity:

> There is a "suspended animation," an impermanence of living the fat body. The act of living fat is itself an act of defiance, an eschewal of discursive modes of bodily being. Seemingly, the fat body exists as a deviant, perverse form of embodiment and, in order to be accorded personhood, is expected to engage in a continual process of transformation, of becoming and, indeed, unbecoming. The process of transformation entails a constant disavowal of one's own flesh. The fat body can only exist (however uncomfortably) as a body aware of its own necessary impermanence. Consequently, in experiencing my fat body there is a sense of suspension, of deferral, of hiatus. One is waiting to become "thin," to become "sexual," waiting to become. (155)

The closet is a place to hide the self. Fat obviously cannot be hidden, but a few women reported feeling like they had to literally hide in their homes. Marissa (34, white) told me that she rarely leaves the house because of the mistreatment and stares she receives when she is in public. She is hiding in her home and "waiting to become" a different person or a different body: one who is not mistreated, who is thin(ner), and who is looked on favorably.

Others remain hidden or "closeted" by distancing themselves from what it means to be fat while they "wait to become" thin. This strategy is paradoxical; they frequently try to distance themselves socially from other fat people, or they mention how incredibly hard it is to accept that they are "one of them," while at the same time they engage in behaviors that perpetuate the stereotypes that many hold about fat people.

I argue that this paradox is best explained by the phenomenon of hyper(in)visibility. The constant attention that is placed on "obesity" by the media, politicians, and the medical community perpetuates the idea that fat is—or should be—a temporary state, because "responsible fat people" should always be trying to lose weight. The majority of women in this study identified with these larger cultural values and have internalized fatphobia—they remain hidden or in the closet. As a result, their enactment of stereotypical behaviors is a reflection of internalized oppression.

Fatphobia and Bullying

During my conversations with these 74 women, there were numerous accounts of harassment from strangers. The verbal abuse they endured was shocking and heartbreaking; I did not expect to hear so many stories of strangers shouting hateful epithets. For example, Linda told me about an incident where a young woman at a public gym said to her, "It's people like you who ruin it for all of us." I responded, "Why do you think she . . . I don't understand." Linda explained:

> I honestly think I triggered . . . obesity triggers fear in other people. It triggers the idea that there is disorder and there is pain. Number one, that someone might get there if they drop their willpower, that that might happen to them. I realize that people's fear of fat and prejudice comes from self, and they can see it happening to them. They look at a fat person like me and they see what could happen to them. I think unfortunately human beings tend to want to feel better about themselves and feel better than other people. We look at people and we compare ourselves—whether it's their income or their whatever—and we say, "Oh, we're better than that or we can be that." (Linda, 40, mixed ethnicity Latina)

Linda made it clear that people do not just hate fat people—they are actually afraid of fat people, because it reminds them that they, too, could become fat. If they react in a hateful or morally superior way, then they can distance themselves from the "shameful" fat person.

Wendy discussed the same idea, that seeing or interacting with a fat person invokes strong reactions from people because they are afraid of becoming fat:

> I would say that there's always going to be a small percentage of people whom, when I deal with them in person, react very strongly against me. Usually it's because I represent something they're afraid of becoming. It's never about me. It's about what's going on in their head . . . I know there's a certain portion of the population that's just going to believe that I am a symbol of what's wrong with America and I can't really help that. I've got to get my damn groceries, you know? I didn't like to have to do that [use the motorized scooter], but after a couple of times of leaving the grocery store without getting what I needed because it hurt so much to be there, I finally succumbed. Now I have the handicap parking sticker and so forth. (Wendy, 47, white)

Wendy is at the heavier end of the weight spectrum, and she indicated that the weight has caused her to have some mobility issues, so she now has to use a motorized scooter because it is too painful for her to walk. She is hypervisible on the scooter and hates it. As she indicates, a fat woman in a motorized scooter signifies to others "how horrible it is to be fat" and symbolizes laziness. She represents "everything that is wrong with America" because it plays into the stereotype that Americans are so "fat and lazy" that they cannot even walk around a grocery store. The emphasis on individual responsibility regarding body size contributes significantly to these stereotypes, and these hateful typecasts frequently turn into harassment and bullying.

Brooke described the harassment she has endured over the course of her life: "I had rocks thrown at me, frog legs thrown at me, constant verbal abuse. Kids tried to beat me up. It was just constant and most of the times teachers would look the other way. It was just a constant, constant stream of, 'You're less than human.' If you're taught your whole life, every day, that you are intrinsically not okay or that you're something that's an object of disgust or revulsion, how does anyone who grew up with that escape that without being totally messed up?" (Brooke, 35, white).

She makes a good point: How is it possible for someone to grow up being treated so horribly and not have some psychological scars to show for the abuse?

Sadly, some of the women I spoke to had previously contemplated or actually attempted suicide as a result of bullying and internalized self-hatred. Consider the predicament of Marilyn: "The bullying because of my size got so bad that I tried to kill myself. There was a juncture in my junior year that I convinced my mother that I wanted to finish school home study and I was able to do it because I found a Home Study School that would do it. I did it mail order, so to speak, and I finished everything early" (Marilyn, 60, white).

The fact that Marilyn was being bullied in the 1960s shows that fatphobia is not a new phenomenon.[4] Fraser (2009) argues that beliefs associated with the virtues of thinness and aversion to fat can be traced back to the economic shifts that took place in the United States in the late 1800s. Industrialization brought ample food supplies and a shift from agriculture to heavy manufacturing. Concurrently, the United States experienced a large influx of Eastern European immigrants who appeared stockier than the previous generation of Western European immigrants. When it became possible for those with modest means to gain weight, it was no longer prestigious to be heavy. Affluent and privileged Americans sought ways to distance themselves from the most recent round of immigrants and to display their social class status. According to Fraser, several disparate factors coalesced that favored thinness—namely, morality, medicine, class status, modernity, women's changing roles, and consumerism. Therefore, thin became chic and symbolized discipline and privilege—the modern woman—whereas fatness symbolized gluttony, immorality, and indigence.

There is a history of treating fat persons as the "less than" or the "inferior" Other, which is why Marilyn's story is unfortunately not unique. Due to the tremendous amount of bullying she experienced and all the pressure she felt to lose weight, she has lived most of her life feeling like she is worthless. She had Lap-Band[5] surgery in Mexico before it was approved in the United States, and she thinks it is the only thing that helped her keep her "weight and appetite under control." Marilyn has experienced a lifetime of surveillance and Othering because of her body size and has made numerous attempts through weight-loss diets to contain her "out-of-control" body. Marilyn says she has a "disorder," which she describes as an inability to become satiated. Before surgery, she was always hungry, but she said her postsurgery appetite is "normal" and she is sated after eating. The Lap-Band has not made her thin, but she has lost enough weight to be at the lower end of the "obese" category (according to BMI). She credits the weight loss with her ability to engage in many of the activities she loves, such as teaching a yoga class.

Bullying and harassment come not only from strangers but also from parents and family. For example, Rochelle, whom I introduced in Chapter 1, reported,

> She would tell me, "You got to quit eating so"—and this would be angry, foul, not a concerned conversation—"You got to quit eating so much, you are going to be as big as a house." That was her catchphrase, "You're going to be big as a house." At 10, 11, 12 it was, "You're going to be a teenager soon, you're going to want a boyfriend and you're not going to have one because of your weight. You're not going to be able to wear the things you want to wear," that kind of stuff. She never said the words, "You are a bad person because you are overweight," but that's definitely the message that came with it. (Rochelle, 35, African American)

Rochelle made it clear that her mother was (and is) devastated by Rochelle's weight. Rochelle is the child of a blended family; her siblings from her mother's first marriage are all thin, and her siblings from her father's first marriage are mostly fat. Rochelle's mother is "beside herself" that Rochelle takes after her father's side and got his "bad genes." Her mother tried to manage Rochelle's weight by telling her that boys would not like her or that she would not have cute clothes to wear, but these threats did not change Rochelle's weight. In fact, in her 20s she gained almost one hundred pounds in a year before she was finally diagnosed with polycystic ovarian syndrome (PCOS).[6] It is possible that her mother's obsession with her body was in part generated from a not-so-subtle concern that Rochelle would suffer socioeconomically for being fat.

Fatness tends to be associated with women of color and the poor. Rochelle's mother may have been concerned that Rochelle would experience downward mobility because of the intersection of her race, body size, and gender. However, the manner in which her mother picked on her and the things she said to her about her own attractiveness has affected Rochelle in adulthood. Rochelle said that she frequently wonders whether her husband is really attracted to her, even though he has never made any indication that her weight is a problem or that he is not attracted to her. She said it is because of the messages she received that fat is ugly. When strangers and loved ones comment on the unsightliness of one's appearance, it is hard not to internalize those feelings and come to accept them as truth.

Bullying and messages about fat hatred also stem from governments and the media. In 2011 and 2012, the state of Georgia launched a Strong4Life campaign to "educate" people about fat and the harms of childhood "obesity."[7] The campaign included television advertisements and billboards with pictures of fat children. Just below each child's picture the word "WARNING" appeared in bold, red, capital letters. Under the word "WARNING" a statement followed, which varied in content depending on the child who was pictured. Some of the statements read, "Fat prevention begins at home. And the buffet line." or "It's hard to be a little girl. If you're not." Critics of the campaign point out that these sorts of public messages actually lead to more harm than good. For instance, research has shown that public shaming does not lead to weight loss or "healthier habits" but instead can lead to weight gain, not to mention that it fuels fatphobia and internalized oppression (Puhl and Heuer 2010; Sutin and Terracciano 2013).

Internalizing Fatphobia: The Looking Glass (Fat) Body

The internalization of fat hatred was an extraordinarily common theme among this sample of women. In Chapter 1, I introduced the concept of the "looking-glass body," which is Waskul and Vannini's (2006) adaptation of Cooley's (1902) "looking-glass self." These concepts stress the importance of reflected perception in the formation of our view of self and body. In essence, we see someone looking at us, and we imagine what this person is thinking about who we are and what we look like. If we experience similar encounters with others, we are much more likely to see ourselves in the manner we imagine most people see us, completing the reflection.

Years of fat hatred, racism, and homophobia impact the way people imagine how others see them, and a few of the women noted similarities in the ways that fat persons and people of color are seen. For instance, Fernanda noted the similarities between racism and sizeism when she was talking about how she has internalized the message that fat is revolting: "I can see now how much I do internalize it, too. I saw something about Jewish people, how a lot of them internalize their racism. I have never thought about it that way. Then I thought that's what overweight people do absolutely. We absolutely internalize it; I think people of other races, like racial minorities do it too, now that I think about it, but it's like you hate yourself, like oh fat people, you know, and then you're one of them" (Fernanda, 36, Latina). She makes it clear that it is the internalization not only of racism but also of sizeism. Fat women of color experience multiple forms of marginalization because they are discriminated against for their race/ethnicity, their gender, and their body (Cross 1991).

According to some scholars, the "war on obesity" may actually be the result of racism and sexism (Boero 2012; Saguy 2013). The hypervisibility of the "obesity epidemic" reinforces shame and guilt fat women feel about who they are and what they look like. "For a long time I, like, would not look at myself in the mirror. You know? I would not even touch my body, really. Especially, like, my belly or my butt, or something like that. I wouldn't touch myself, because I was afraid, if you touch yourself that'll make it real. You know? If you don't see it and you don't feel it, maybe it's not really there" (Karen, 24, white). Karen revealed that she avoided touching her body to distance herself from her fat. If she could feel the fat on her body then she felt like she had to admit that she is fat and being fat means, culturally anyway, that one is less than or inferior. Jessica said, "This may be overblown, but it is a relatively accurate depiction of my fears. I look at my whole life, and it scares me how deeply this current of self-hatred runs in me. I am tired of it, it exhausts me, I don't want it anymore, but it is as familiar as the proverbial old pair of slippers, and some part of me clings to it like a baby blanket" (Jessica, 35, white). Jessica wants to overcome the feelings she has of self-hatred, but she makes it clear that this is incredibly difficult because she identifies with the larger cultural views about the harms of fat, which fuels fatphobia outwardly and inwardly.

Numerous scholars and activists argue that the "war on obesity" has increased the discrimination and mistreatment of people of size. For instance, research has shown that as the media emphasis and attention on "obesity" has heightened, so has the amount of prejudice and discrimination reported by fat persons (Puhl and Heuer 2010).

Because of the association in the scholarship between the media focus on "obesity" and fat hatred, I asked the women what they thought about the attention that was being paid to the "obesity epidemic":

> You know it's really easy for me to point and say, "I'm not that." And then, over the last almost seven years, I am that. And, you know, what does that say about me? It says I'm a loser. And so when people start talking about the epidemics and people being overweight and not wanting to pay for somebody's bad health because they don't take care of themselves, and I can't chime into that. I can't have a voice there. Because I'm in that category of people they're talking about. So I don't have the right to comment on certain things until I can get to a different place. (Patricia, 47, white)

Patricia attempts to distance herself from other fat people but then concedes that she is now "one of them." Her language makes it clear that being fat is something "less than"; she says she is "a loser" because she is fat. In fact, she goes on to state that because she is a "fat loser," she has no voice in the debate about the "obesity epidemic." She seems to think that those who are affected most—those labeled "obese"—do not deserve a voice in the conversation about weight and health.

Sue, a 62-year-old Canadian, spoke with me about the pressure she has felt over the years from her family, her lovers, and herself to lose weight. She said that many of the men she has been romantically involved with focused on her weight. One partner in particular frequently called her a pig and other hurtful names.[8] "The minute he would say that, I could feel my shoulders going down and I wanted to sink into the ground and think, 'He's so right. I am such a pig.'" I asked her if she really believed that, if she believed that she was a "pig," and she said she did. Sue's perception of herself was that she was lazy, stupid, and a "pig" because she "couldn't get it together to lose weight." She internalized the messages from the larger culture about why people are fat and also the abuse she received from her significant other. Sue went on to discuss the cultural messages about fat and how it has impacted her views of herself and other fat people:

> *Sue:* "Oh, my God, she is so pretty, why doesn't she lose weight?" "Oh, my God, what a slob." "Oh my God, her pants are so tight." "Oh my God, she's killing herself." "Look at that woman over there eating a chocolate bar instead of a carrot stick. Doesn't she see what she looks like?" "I would never date a fat girl." You know, society can be cruel.
> *JG:* Yeah, absolutely. Sometimes it is hard not to internalize those messages.
> *Sue:* Definitely. To be honest with you, I have those thoughts myself about other people. (Sue, 62, white)

Most were embarrassed to admit it, but numerous women told me that they, too, hold other fat people in low regard. Sophia, a 55-year-old white woman, said, "I mean I'm guilty of this myself. I'm fat, but I will look at a fat person sometimes and have feelings like that. I hate that part of myself. I don't like that part of myself." Sophia, Sue, and Patricia not only hated their own bodies and selves for being fat but also hated other fat people. This may be surprising for some, but it is consistent with other research that has shown that fat individuals tend to hold antifat attitudes, though they are generally less severe than those of their thinner peers (Crandall 1994; Schwartz et al. 2006).

As Kyrölä (2005, 99) states, "Fatness becomes a closet of fear, a dangerous shell that prevents the real person (woman) inside from being and being seen as her 'true' petite self." As a society, we assume that people who are fat are fat because they overeat and do not exercise, but there also seems to be an irrational fear that "fat is contagious." In her memoir, *Read My Hips*, Kim Brittingham (2011) describes an informal "experiment" that she conducted on public buses in New York City. She created a mock book jacket with the title *Fat Is Contagious: How Sitting Next to a Fat Person*

Can Make You Fat, wrapped it around a real book, and read it while on the bus. She was prompted to make the book cover because of the frequent sneers directed at her on the bus because of her size. When she read from the fictitious book on the bus, people literally got up and moved away from her, strained their necks to read and reread the cover to be sure they saw it correctly, or sat with their mouths open in pure shock and disgust and looked horrified (180). Brittingham's informal "experiment" demonstrates the intense and irrational fear most people have of becoming fat. Due to fears of fat embedded in the culture, those who are fat often feel like they "stand out" in the world in a socially oppressive way. In other words, they are hypervisible.

Liz, a first-year college student, explained to me how difficult it is to be fat on a campus where the majority of the students are thin and fit. She feels like she "stands out" and has been trying to lose weight by modifying her eating habits and exercising at the student recreation center.

> I get more tired a lot quicker than most people do obviously, and I definitely don't like going to the gym because there are a lot of people in-shape there. I feel like one of the main questions when I'm working out is, you know, people look at me, and they'll be like, "Why are you even here trying?" It's so hard because it's like don't judge a book by its cover, but I'm always judging people because I think that they're judging me—when they're probably not. I have to defend myself from people, which is dumb, because I mean they're probably not even worried about me. (Liz, 19, white)

It is interesting that she begins by saying that it is "obvious" that she gets more tired than most people. I asked her why that should be obvious, and she told me it is because she is fat, which to her means she is out of shape and unhealthy.[9] Liz is in the marching band at her university, has a job, is a full-time student, and has no health problems, but she believes that she is unhealthy and "obviously" more tired than others because she is fat. She has internalized the messages from the larger culture that it is impossible to be fat and healthy. Because she believes she is "unhealthy," she is trying to cut her caloric intake and exercise, but exercise is difficult because she feels that her body is on display at the gym. Intellectually, Liz knows that other students at the gym are probably not paying attention to her, but she cannot help feeling like she is constantly subjected to the judgmental gaze of her peers. Karen (24, white) said something very similar when she was talking about her job: "Now, working with the [democratic] party, I feel totally judged every day. It's all very powerful men in there and I'm very much treated like the secretary and I don't think that they necessarily care that I'm unattractive, but that that's kind of a stopping point. You know? That there is no temptation there, 'We'll hire the fat girl. She'll do whatever we ask her to do.' You know? And it's a boys club. I'm the only woman out of a staff of about 20 people."

Karen assumes that she was hired because the men in the office thought she would do work that a thinner (more attractive) woman would not, and that as a bonus, they would not be tempted to have an affair with her because she is fat (unattractive). Karen sees herself as unattractive and thus assumes that others do, too. Both Karen and Liz assume that others see them through the lens of the "stereotypical fat women"—unattractive, out of shape, and out of place. The fact that both Liz and Karen see themselves through the stereotypes of the larger culture shows how pervasive those messages actually are. Liz's and Karen's stories demonstrate the insidiousness of the phenomenon of hyper(in)visibility. They both feel that they are paid a tremendous amount of attention through the judgment of others, while they are both simultaneously erased.

It is not just about attractiveness or physical fitness, though; it is also about how one is treated by others, and many women felt that if they were thinner their lives would be easier. Sara (28, white) said, "It completely goes to people would treat you better, you know. Life in society would be easier if you lost weight, which I think is harder to combat because it's probably true ... But on the whole, you know, oh, people would be nicer to you, and things would be—it would be easier to kind of navigate in this world if you weren't coming up against this prejudice." Sara is trying to fight back against the predominant cultural messages, but she thinks that if she were thinner she would experience less mistreatment. As Janet (26, white) stated, "Well, I never had a problem with somebody like calling me fat to my face or anything like that, but I've often felt inferior, like people look down on me, because of my size."

To be fat is to be inferior, and it is communicated through the real or perceived discriminating gaze of others. These messages bellow from the stranger who shouts sizeist epithets, it comes from the family physician who emphasizes the dangers of fat, and it stems from the media who continually remind us all how harmful/ugly/embarrassing/disgusting it is to be fat. It is nearly impossible to avoid internalizing those messages. This is partly why the phenomenon of hyper(in)visibility is so important to uncover and understand. The combination of sensationalistic attention and public scorn creates a situation where fat women are erased and no longer treated with dignity and respect. The internalization of that lack of dignity and respect perpetuates "doing fat," whereby fat women engage in stereotypical behaviors, and simultaneously influences the structure of the self and one's identity.

Reflected Acts

Phenomenologically, one *becomes* fat by engaging in behaviors that signify fatness, or what I call "doing fat." As I discussed in Chapter 1, "doing fat" comes from West and Zimmerman's (1987) notion of "doing gender" and from West and Fenstermaker's (1995) concept of "doing difference." West and Zimmerman clearly articulated the process by which one becomes gendered. They argue that doing gender is a symbolic accomplishment: it is an emergent feature of social situations. Doing gender is not inherent within the individual, and while it is individuals who do gender, it is a situated doing.

Analogously, I argue that doing fat is also a symbolic accomplishment that emerges in social interactions. Individuals do gender when they organize their activities to reflect or express gender and, in addition, are predisposed to see others' behaviors similarly (West and Zimmerman 1987, 127).

Doing fat also means that fat persons organize their actions to reflect or express being fat and see other fat persons likewise. When the negative connotations associated with fat are internalized, women sometimes act according to those preconceived notions. One of the ways some of these women performed fat was by allowing men to take advantage of them:

> And I had a couple of guys that did that, but I just hated it, and in my life, I haven't been very proactive about, I'd say, protecting my body in that respect. Someone else might be "get the hell off

me, you son of a bitch!" But I've been way too passive about it, because it's a low self-esteem thing. You know? And you feel like for some reason, you deserve to be treated badly. It's weird, but those things—and then the other thing was really just a matter of—the reason I don't exercise as much as I used to is because in the past when I've been out exercising, I've had people scream at me, like just scream at me "you fat bitch," "you fat slut!" One time I was canoeing in the lake and somebody screamed out "why are you so fat?" I was canoeing in the middle of the freakin' lake. And those types of things also kind of happen. We were talking about how it affects people and how you feel about people. And really, over the last four years, I've gone outside less and less because of things like that. (Marissa, 34, white)

I'm okay with talking about it. It doesn't bother me much anymore. I think part of what happened was that I didn't—I think when you're fat, and I think when you're a woman, you have more of a tendency to not have good boundaries. And I think that's part of what happened. I didn't know that—I literally didn't know that I was supposed to have boundaries and that I could say no. (Tina, 34, white)

Both Marissa and Tina emphasize that it was their size, lack of confidence, and low self-esteem that led them to feel like they deserved mistreatment. Marissa "does fat" by removing herself from society. She has practically imprisoned herself in her home, because she cannot deal with the negative attention she receives in public. However, removing herself from the gaze of others further marginalizes her, because she is isolated and is now literally not seen. Moreover, both Marissa (at the beginning of the quote) and Tina talked about the way men have treated them and said that they stayed in those relationships because they did not have boundaries. Neither of them "owned" their bodies. Their bodies not only were separate from them but also belonged to the men in their life. Their purpose was to satisfy these men, not themselves, and they were rendering their needs invisible (I talk more about sex and relationships in Chapter 5)—in this manner, they were engaging in the act of doing fat.

Spatial Discrimination

Public spaces, such as restaurants, medical facilities, classrooms, and so forth, can create unique issues for those who are at the heavier end of the weight spectrum. Chairs with arms are often too narrow, booths in restaurants typically do not provide ample space between the seat and the table, and some seating might not be sturdy enough to accommodate a heavier person. Owen (2012) examined the effects of living as a fat person in a thin world, or what she calls the effect of spatial discrimination. She conceptualized spatial discrimination as the "small and persistent ways that fat bodies are physically derided within our environments" (294). Her participants noted the various ways in which their bodies were ignored or dismissed in public spaces because they physically could not fit in chairs or on public transportation.

Owen (2012) argues that the lack of accommodations for persons of size in public spaces like restaurants, shopping centers, or public transportation constitutes a type of microaggression. A microaggression refers to behaviors or situations that communicate subtle harms or discrimination committed against persons for their race, ethnicity, gender, sexuality, or ability status. Owen states, "[Microaggressions are] a small nibbling at fat persons' sense of worth, a constant wearing down as a result of small but continuous experiences of not fitting, of feeling embarrassed, of having to demand accommodations or else not receive them at all. It's a smaller, less obvious form of violence, but it has many of the same effects: anger, frustration, guilt, fear, and loathing (toward self and/or others)" (295). Numerous women I interviewed talked about the anxiety they endured when they would try a new restaurant or doctor's office. It is humiliating to arrive at a location and not be able to fit, or worse yet to have a chair collapse in public, but it is also embarrassing to have to explain to friends or coworkers, especially if they are not fat, that some public spaces cannot accommodate one's size. Cassie exemplifies that here:

> Yeah. I mean they were like my best friends, I'd known them for years, they knew everything about me, but it was just something I was too embarrassed to say and when I finally would get up the courage and I told a friend, she was like, "Why in the hell didn't you tell me that?" And I was just like, I was just so embarrassed, I didn't

want to bring attention to myself. I didn't want to point out the incredibly obvious fact that I was fat, I mean it was just ridiculous the amount of pain I put myself in just to appear, quote "normal." (Cassie, 33, white)

Cassie is "covering"—a term Goffman (1963) employs to describe situations where the stigmatized individual attempts to minimize her stigmatized status to make "normal" people feel more comfortable. Cassie dismissed her own needs in order to avoid identifying as fat and bringing attention to her body, despite the fact that she told me that she was incredibly uncomfortable and often bruised from squeezing into booths.

Many of the women who endured physical pain, verbal abuse, microaggressions, or other forms of mistreatment saw themselves as deserving of punishment for not losing weight. The pain served as symbolic proof that they did not belong. Cassie eventually told her friends, but she also said that she was not going out as much as she used to because, like Marissa, she could not handle the stares and attention she drew. Plus, she said that she felt bad that her friends had to avoid certain establishments because of her. She felt it was easier if she extracted herself from the situation so that she did not hamper their evening (cf. Owen 2012).

Nicole addresses similar, but distinct, issues with entering new spaces:

> I feel like when I go into any new situation I have to be cognizant of the fact that I'm fat and that carries a lot of morality . . . that carries a lot of connotations about who I am as a person. I feel like I'm cognizant of that issue in almost all situations, like any time I'm going out for drinks to a bar, or when I'm going to a meeting with people, I feel like there's always this part of me that thinks, "What do they think about my body? Do they think I'm incompetent because of my body? Do they think that I'm lazy or unattractive because of my body?" I feel like that's something that . . . You know, almost any group that historically has that sort of moral weight to their body feels when they enter a room like that, especially if it's clear . . . like people with disabilities, or people with different racial backgrounds, people who . . . I know it's not apples-to-apples, I know it's not, but I think that that same sort of stereotype threat exists for fat people and I feel very aware of that whenever I'm entering a new situation. (Nicole, 25, white)

Nicole feels like she is "on stage," similar to Liz who felt she "stood out" on her mostly thin university campus, when she is in public because of her body. She knows that being fat renders her morally inferior in the eyes of many, but the fact that she becomes acutely concerned about the way others see her shows how strong the messages about fat are—she is hypervisible. Doing fat and experiencing the effects of hypervisibility are what Shawna refers to as a "fat girl mentality":

> I've noticed myself, if I'm making something for a potluck, I still fall back under the fat girl mentality. Remember when the actress that was on *The Practice*—what was her name, the fat girl? I forgot her name. Anyway, I remember watching on *Inside Edition* or something one night, she was talking about being a fat girl and how Hollywood . . . She walks on her first day on set at *The Practice* and they had her desk set up on the set, and they had a candy dish. She said, "Hell no, this fat girl has a candy dish on her desk. That's way too stereotypical. We put that in our drawer." [laughter] I'm like, "I still do that." Because if they say, "Could you make a meal for so and so," I'm like, "Oh God, what am I going to make?" Because if I make something . . . I think a new mom should have something really yummy. She needs the calories. (Shawna, 34, white)

Shawna was worried that if she made something with too much fat in it then people would judge her because she is a fat woman. She feels like others police her behaviors, especially those related to food. She does fat by second-guessing herself, and she struggles to think of something to cook that will not out her as a fat person. She mentioned that it is a challenge, because she fears that if she makes something too healthy or low-calorie, then people will think she is doing it because she is fat, but if she makes something that is too rich or calorie dense, then it will provide people with "proof" of why Shawna is fat. She knows that it is absurd to think this way, hence the reason she calls it "fat girl mentality," but it is difficult not to slip into these familiar thought patterns.

As Shawna's case clearly indicates, most of these women are aware that they engage in behaviors that are stereotypical of fat women, and they work hard to avoid perpetuating those beliefs. One of the ways that numerous women attempted to overcome the perpetuation of the "fat girl mentality" was through demonstrating or proclaiming that they are more than a body.

More than a Fat Woman

Strikingly, many of the women I interviewed talked about their bodies as separate from their self or mind. The conception of the mind as a separate, distinct entity from the body, with the rational mind as superior to the irrational body, continues to infuse common discourse and self-conception. Such a distinction, between the self and body, reflects deeply seated conceptions of humans that have a long history in sundry cultures, particularly in the Western tradition, as in Descartes's argument for a mind/body dualism, the view that the mind or soul is metaphysically distinct from the body. According to this Cartesian picture, the immaterial rational mind is the seat of free will and is superior to the irrational emotional body, which is the seat of desire. Such dualism reflects the cultural preoccupation with a soul in the Judeo-Christian tradition and continues to exist as a part of many Westerners' worldview and influences how they conceive of themselves—"young at heart" or "mentally strong" are common statements that emphasize the separation of mind and body.

In addition to the dominant cultural framing of a mind/body split, it is common for those who are Othered and part of a stigmatized group to want to remove themselves, at least symbolically, from association with deviant characteristics. Numerous women said things to suggest that they are more than their body. I heard repeatedly, "I'm smart, I work hard, but I just happen to be fat." Or they would say, as Ann (33, white) did, "I mean, it's a part of who I am. It affects who I am. But it's not the only thing I am." Ann makes it clear that being fat affects her, but that she is so much more than her body. She does not want to claim a fat identity because it is only one aspect of herself and she feels that she would be the same person regardless of her body size.

Krista discusses a similar issue but employs it to boost her view of herself and to explain why she has "decent self-esteem":

> Because even at the weight I'm at now, it sounds like such a big number and I mean it is a big number but I don't feel like I'm . . . like when you say oh that person weighs 270 pounds, I don't know too many people that could look at me and say oh you weigh 270 pounds because our perception is different. I don't know and I think that's part of maybe why I have a decent self-esteem, because

> I don't look at myself and go, oh you're 200 and something pounds or whatever, I look at myself as a person and . . . I don't know. (Krista, 28, white)

The fact that Krista feels like she is an exception to have "decent self-esteem" at 270 pounds also indicates the power of the messages that women hear. It is abnormal for women—especially fat women—to have decent self-esteem, because they are told that their value is tied to their appearance.

Naomi Wolf ([1991] 2002), in her book *The Beauty Myth*, argues that the idea that beauty is objective and universal is a myth. She contends that beauty is a system of currency created by politics to maintain men's dominance and power. In fact, beauty is not about appearance; it is about prescribing behavior. Youth, thinness, and virginity are prized and deemed beautiful because they symbolize women's lack of power. Women who are young are not yet powerful or knowledgeable, those who are thin are weak, and those who are virginal are inexperienced; in essence, these women do not threaten the social order.

Wolf ([1991] 2002) asserts that the beauty myth is the modern day iron maiden, a medieval torture device. The iron maiden was a casket with a beautiful, smiling woman painted on the outside, but the inside of the casket was lined with steel spikes that caused the victim to slowly bleed to death. Wolf argues that the strictures prescribed by the beauty myth are similarly rigid, cruel, and euphemistically painted. Moreover, the prescriptions for beauty over time have become increasingly narrow and difficult to achieve, which leads to a state of "normative discontent" or perpetual bodily dissatisfaction: "I'm trying to accept myself. The way I am, the way I look. I'm trying to think of myself not so much in terms of my weight as defining who I am, but I think I'm . . . I'm an outgoing person, I have a good sense of humor, I think I'm pretty funny sometimes, and so I'm trying to focus more on those attributes than just my weight" (Mandy, 32, white).

Mandy's language clearly demonstrates what Wolf ([1991] 2002) was writing about. She is *trying* to accept herself and the way she looks, but she cannot seem to find bodily acceptance because her fat body does not represent conventional beauty. In an effort to feel better about herself, she attempts to symbolically distance who she is—her sense of humor and personality—from her "deviant body." She reminds herself that she is more than her body; she is a fun person. Elizabeth also demonstrates this mentality:

> I'll take on a lot more projects so I can prove my worth that, "See, even though I'm big I'm valuable to your company." Also having confidence in my abilities helps a lot to substitute that I'm feeling lacking physically or visually. I'm very smart. I'm very logical. I get things done. I can produce outcomes in any way, shape, or form. Whether that was doing karate when I was younger, or softball, or whatever, I was able to be on the winning team. I could be the winning one. That can also counterbalance. If I'm not maybe what you need physically, I'm still going to be awesome mentally. So, I can be good in the personality aspect. That helps me confidence-wise. (Elizabeth, 30, white)

Elizabeth takes on more work because she is "visually lacking," and she feels like she must prove to her employer that despite her looks she is more than a fat person because she is intelligent, logical, and can get the task accomplished. For Elizabeth, emphasizing her abilities and personality helps her maintain her confidence.

Many who promote Health at Every Size® or other body-positive messages stress the notion that all people are more than their body, the size of their jeans, or the number on the scale. Parents frequently tell their children, "It's what's on the inside that matters," and while those messages are powerful and should be true, it is tremendously difficult to get along in society if one's body is visually obtrusive. It was reassuring to see that there were a number of women with whom I spoke who were or are currently trying to embody this notion and find self-acceptance, but unfortunately they are the exception and not the rule when it comes to women's views of their own bodies.

Conclusion

Throughout this chapter, I have demonstrated the ways in which the women I interviewed negotiated fatphobia and internalized oppression. The embodiment of self-hatred led many to engage in behaviors that perpetuate stereotypes about fat persons, fat women in particular. I also demonstrated that because of the stigma associated with fat, fatphobia, and internalized oppression, many also sought to symbolically distance themselves from a fat self, identity, and their own fat bodies. They employed numerous techniques to demonstrate to others that they are more than their body, which is typically symbolic of excess and irresponsibility.

Fat tends to be associated with the poor and with persons of color, whereas thinness tends to be associated with privilege, higher social status, and conspicuous leisure. Some scholars have argued that the association between fat, the poor, and racial and ethnic minorities explains the heightened attention and hostility toward "obesity" (Boero 2012; Saguy 2013). In this respect, the "war on obesity" is another mechanism to enact control over the bodies of women and people of color. In a neoliberal state, it is everyone's responsibility to be "healthy," and because fat is framed as unhealthy, those who are fat are subject to increasing surveillance and social control.

The phenomenon of hyper(in)visibility explains the complicated ways in which these women see their bodies and selves and form their identities. Some of them expressed fears about becoming fat or seeing themselves as fat, and they implied that they are waiting to become thin. Hyper(in)visibility works to reinforce the internalization of fatphobia and oppression. These women reported that they experience overt discrimination and mistreatment from strangers, peers, and even loved ones because of their body size. When the state gets involved, such as with Georgia's Strong4Life campaign, fatphobia is reinforced and sanctioned. Perpetual mistreatment, microaggressions, and hypervisibility lead many of these women to attempt to distance their self from their body. They try to make it clear that they are different than other fat people, but it often results in them seeing their selves and bodies through the judgmental eyes of others. Such an identification of the self manifests itself in their behaviors. Some of the women talked about trying to make themselves socially invisible by not leaving the house or by spending little time in public spaces.

The phenomenon of hyper(in)visibility perpetuates the stigma and negative stereotypes commonly associated with fat people, because some of them "do fat" or act in a manner that is consistent with society's expectations about fat women. They may fail to establish boundaries, render their own needs or desires invisible, or believe they deserve mistreatment or punishment because they are fat. For instance, they take on the "fat girl mentality" or they fail to establish boundaries in intimate relationships.

Numerous women wanted it to be known that they are more than fat persons. They were not necessarily closeted about their fatness nor were they coming out as fat. What their comments suggest is that their personalities, intelligence, feelings, and so forth are more important than their body size and that they want to be acknowledged for more than their bodies. They were concerned that their identity not be wrapped up in "being a fat person" because they are more than that, and they feel that even if they were not fat that they would still be the same person. In Chapter 6, I highlight the experiences of women who have come out as fat and embody fat as an identity.

Fatphobia and internalized oppression can lead to harmful behaviors such as suicide or suicide attempts, disregarding one's needs and physical comforts, and even—as we will see in Chapter 3—excessive dieting and sometimes dangerous weight-loss behaviors. Social isolation and perpetual stress can also lead to physiological problems such as depression, hypertension, and heart disease. Subverting the dominant discourse can lead to body- and self-acceptance, as we will see in Chapter 6, but it is a hard road to travel—especially without support.

Chapter 3

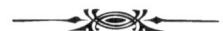

Fixing the Fat Body

The abject is the realm of "I don't want to be that!" (Butler 1993, 3). Butler describes the abject body as the material body that has smeared or blurred symbolic borders. The fat body is abject and hyper(in)visible. It is considered grotesque, it is loathed, and many go to extreme measures to eradicate it. It is stereotyped as out of control, and frequently its mere presence poses a threat to the self, the scene of interaction, and to others who must interact with "It."

Abjection is important for understanding participants' internalization of fat hatred and attempts to rid their bodies of fat. Essentially, abjection is characterized by fear of contamination and revulsion; it is set in the past, but it is always in the forefront of one's thoughts (Kristeva 1982). In a fatphobic society, people fear that they will become fat, and the sight of fat bodies disgusts them. As we saw in Chapter 2, those who are fat typically attempt to dissociate fat from their selves and/or identities, meaning they distance themselves from the negative stereotypes associated with fat or they view their corpulence as temporary. For many who lose weight, the fear of regaining it is omnipresent as are the attempts to lose it or expel it.

This chapter focuses on three main issues. First, I discuss how others—strangers, physicians, teachers, and family members—attempt to manage participants' bodies. Second, I explore how participants police their own bodies and employ a variety of tools to "fix" their abject bodies. And third, I highlight the 26 participants who quit both dieting and trying to change their bodies, despite the pressure to do so.

As we saw in Chapter 2, these women tended to talk about their bodies as separate from their selves or minds. By discussing their bodies and minds as separate entities, they are able to symbolically distance who they are from the stereotypes that many hold about fat people. However, the mind/body split contributes to self-objectification and hyper(in)visibility when fat women see their bodies as abject or as objects of revulsion—something separate from the *real* them. Dieting, exercise, and weight-loss surgery serve as tools to liberate the self from the abject fat.

Participants' experiences traversing numerous diets, engagement in disordered eating behaviors, and weight-loss surgery illustrate the expectations others have about what they should or should not do with their bodies and their own struggles with their body image and acceptance of self. Nearly all these women were expected from a young age to "fix" their "unsightly" body; in essence, they were implored to lose weight.

Due to the stigma and marginalization associated with "obesity," fat women's bodies are highly visible but rarely seen (Tischner 2013). As I discussed Chapter 1, the phenomenon of hyper(in)visibility exists on a continuum. At one extreme, fat bodies are paid a tremendous amount of attention through the media, government agencies, or medicine because of the physical presence of a large body. At the other extreme, fat bodies are frequently erased, ignored, or nonexistent in social interactions, on television or in movies, by physicians, and in other public and private spaces. Hyper(in)visibility is a mode of Othering that occurs at both the structural and experiential levels; it is also an embodied performance that takes place in social situations.

OTHERS' ATTEMPTS TO CONTAIN, FIX, AND MANAGE PARTICIPANTS' ABJECT BODIES

One of the ways that hyper(in)visibility manifests itself in the lives of large women is through how they are treated in public spaces—especially restaurants, grocery stores, and when eating in public. Numerous women mentioned the fact that they frequently felt like they should order less food (or less fattening foods) when they are at a restaurant because they were concerned with being judged. Shawna, whom I introduced in Chapter 2, referred to this as "fat girl mentality." This fat girl mentality puts them in a double bind, because if they order "diet food," they feel like people think, "She must be trying to lose weight." If they order a hamburger and French fries or a cream sauce, they feel like people are thinking, "No wonder she's so fat, if she eats like that." Of course, ordering a salad or a low-fat meal may have nothing to do with dieting, and eating a hamburger or a calorie-dense dish does not make someone fat—plenty of thin people eat hamburgers and cream sauce, but because of thin privilege it goes unnoticed.

Several women reported that they have caught other customers in restaurants staring at them, and a few actually had strangers approach them and comment on what they were eating. There were also five women who told me stories about walking down the street in a large city eating an ice cream cone or street food, and they were subjected to people shouting at them about how they should "quit eating" or "stop stuffing their fat faces."

Women also talked about how highly visible they felt in grocery stores. Many reported that they feel like everyone is watching them and judging their food choices—especially women who have mobility problems and use the in-store mobility scooters. Several women told me that they have had people make comments about the contents of their grocery carts and have seen people shake their heads in disapproval. Given how frequently fat women are mistreated in public, many were extremely sensitive to even the most subtle stares or looks of disgust (cf. Tischner 2013). These experiences lead to feelings of being constantly under the microscope, which in turn perpetuates their own self-discipline and surveillance (Foucault 1977).

One of the most prominent themes that emerged during my conversations with participants who have been large their whole life was that from a young age they were told that their bodies were unacceptable and in need of "being fixed." Between the ages of 8 and 12, parents, teachers, peers, and physicians started encouraging, suggesting, or demanding that interviewees lose weight. Participants who have been large their whole life became aware early on that being fat, or even chubby, was a problem, and that they would likely suffer serious social and health consequences as a result. Rachel (26, white) said, "It wasn't necessarily outwardly negative so much as it was just sort of this attitude that

I needed to be fixed or I was doing something wrong, some of my teachers would take me aside and talk to me, and ask me what was going on, and my fifth grade teacher talked me into working out with him after school a few days a week, and people made an effort to change me, and nothing ever worked, so what can you do?" Rachel said she started gaining weight "rapidly" when she was nine, and that "everyone was trying to figure out what was wrong." Her parents, pediatrician, and teachers told her to stop eating so much and failed to believe her when she said she was not overeating. Her body became visibly larger, and the adults in her life assumed that it was because she ate too much, which is part of the popular discourse surrounding weight gain. The adults instilled in her that it was not normal to be large and that it was a problem. They seemed to discount that the weight gain might be due to genetics, a metabolic condition, or possibly that Rachel is naturally at the larger end of the weight spectrum. The cultural messages about the problems with fat and how one becomes fat are so strong that there is no other explanation except overeating and lack of exercise. Samantha Murray refers to these cultural meanings as "collective knowingness" (Murray 2005, 1562). In other words, we as a society believe that we know a fat person's habits just from looking at the person.

A few weeks before Rachel spoke with me, she was diagnosed with polycystic ovarian syndrome (PCOS) and hypothyroidism (both contribute to weight gain).[1] It is not clear if those conditions caused the weight gain at age nine, but what is clear is that she has struggled with her self-esteem and confidence because of her size. She discussed feeling down because a recent surgery and new medications caused her to gain some weight. She told me that she has had to work hard to gain the confidence she has, and now that she can be active again, she is hoping to regain some of that confidence, partly through losing weight. Those early messages about having an unacceptable body continue to haunt her today.

Messages from teachers or doctors about being too fat were not taken lightly or forgotten. In fact, many of the women were able to recall those events or conversations in painstaking detail. For example, Carol told me,

> I went to the doctor with a sore throat. I was in fifth grade. This doctor comes in, he looks at me, and he starts screaming, and I'm not

exaggerating here, screaming about my size, that I already weigh as much as he does, and that I'm going to die of a heart attack by the time I'm 30. And I'm 30 now, and no heart attacks, knock on wood. But like he—I couldn't believe this guy, and he's like poking my stomach, like he's giving me an examination, and he's poking my stomach, and my mom starts talking about my grades and how I'm so smart, and I swear to God he said, "Don't tell me she's smart. If she was smart, she wouldn't be this fat." (Carol, 30, white)

The fact that her physician behaved in this manner and implied that fat people are not smart is appalling, but unfortunately she was not the only participant to experience this sort of treatment from a family physician. Three participants revealed that they had been prescribed amphetamines for weight loss during adolescence! That their physicians thought it was appropriate to prescribe amphetamines to a young girl reflects the general view of fatness: Fat is abject, and possible addiction or health problems as a result of amphetamine use is negligible compared to fatness.[2]

Family members used a variety of tools to "inspire" participants to lose weight. The following quote from Pam about her mother illustrates the pressure she felt to change or fix her body: "She's always like—she was always the one to, when I was a kid, put me on diets. At 10 years old, she put me on Nutrisystem and I dieted on and off until I was about 20. And when I got older and could make my own decisions, she was always super eager to have me diet or work out. She would really overly support that—always seemed like she wanted to change me" (Pam, 29, white). It was not just Pam's mother who wanted to change her; Pam reported that she does not like to visit doctors because they always comment on her weight, even if her ailment has nothing to do with her weight. She said that a recent visit with her primary care physician ended with him telling her she should consider lap band (a type of weight-loss surgery). When she said she did not think that it was healthy, he agreed with her, but still thought she should have the procedure. Pam's mother and her doctors perceive her fat as abject—something that is revolting and needs to be expelled. Even if it involves a procedure that the physician deems unhealthy, it is better than being fat.[3]

Women reported experiencing contempt, ridicule, and monetary manipulation from family members to fix their bodies. In the next excerpt, Miranda talks about losing more than one hundred pounds on a "suicide diet." She called it a "suicide diet" because she was restricting her caloric intake to the point of near starvation:

> The reason why I started that diet was actually because of a conversation with my mom. When I came to the US for my PhD, I gained weight. I was already too heavy and I gained 30 pounds. My mom told me that if I didn't lose weight I was going to have to have surgery. It wasn't a question or a suggestion, and even though I was 29 or 30 at the time, yes, my mom does make that type of decisions for me. She was in a position, or she is and always has been, in a position that I would have let her make that decision for me. (Miranda, 34, Latina)

Miranda's mother gave her an ultimatum: lose weight or have weight-loss surgery. Miranda explained that there is tremendous pressure for women in the Dominican Republic to meet the conventional beauty standards. She said that even though she has earned her doctorate, the most important thing to her family was how big or small she was and whether she had a boyfriend.

I asked Miranda how the Dominican Republic compared to the United States regarding the attention paid to "obesity." She said that in the Dominican Republic people are much more outspoken about telling someone they are fat or that they need to lose weight. She perceived the United States as more tolerant of fat and felt that most people are fairly covert when it comes to fatphobia.

It was fairly common for interviewees to share stories about how their families used money to inspire weight loss: "Well, my mother was concerned, and she was always like if I lost five or ten pounds or something, she would give me money. That would be like her reward if I was able to lose some weight, she'd give me money" (Janet, 36, white). Janet reported that the weight loss "never stuck," if she lost any weight at all. Other women talked about their parents offering to pay them to exercise, such as running up and down a steep, long driveway multiple times, or offering to buy them clothes if they lost weight. The fact that so many parents were so invested in their daughter's weight reveals a lot about societal views of fat—it is abject and must be expelled.

The policing of large women's bodies comes from many sources and is a component of the phenomenon of hyper(in)visibility.

According to a study about youths (both boys and girls) and weight-based victimization (i.e., psychological and/or physiological mistreatment), perpetrators were most commonly peers (92 percent) and friends (70 percent), followed by adult perpetrators, including physical education teachers / sport coaches (42 percent), parents (37 percent), and teachers (27 percent; Puhl, Peterson, and Luedicke 2012). The stories from the women I interviewed indicated a very similar trend, except that the women I spoke with seemed to report higher levels of weight-based victimization from parents, in addition to grandparents, siblings, and extended family. It is likely that these women experienced higher levels of victimization than those in the Puhl et al. study because this is a gendered phenomenon—there is more pressure on women to meet the conventional standard of beauty than there is for men.

Claire and Cassie both discussed how their fathers influenced their body image:

> I didn't gain weight until [my] midteens, and it wasn't even that I gained a lot of weight, but in my mind, I was fat and went on Weight Watchers. And since then, kind of a binge eating cycle started, so at my heaviest point, my Dad would say stuff like oh—he'd kind of make sarcastic comments. Like oh, "move your fat ass." Or "look at the size of you." And it's not only him commenting on me, but like commenting on other family members, so you know that that's his feelings toward people who are overweight. (Claire, 35, white)

> My first memory, I was four-years-old, my father took me into the bathroom and taught me how to make myself throw up. And he told me that if I did it I wouldn't get fat; and if I did get fat nobody would love me. (Cassie, 33, white)

Both Claire and Cassie suffered weight-based victimization from their fathers, and while the majority of cases were not as severe as Cassie's, there were numerous reports from participants about parents shaming them, teasing them, and bullying them about their weight.

Women, fat or not, are taught from a young age about the importance of appearance. As several women's mothers or grandmothers frequently lamented, "You have such a pretty face; if only you would lose weight." Thinness is equated with beauty and health, and for most it requires substantial effort, not to mention the unrelenting supervision and commentary from others when one is not thin:

> My mother was really concerned about our weight, so she pretty much starved us throughout our whole early childhood. Nothing with fat in it pretty much ever crossed our household. She was very into natural foods. And so I wasn't very heavy as a child, but I was constantly under scrutiny. I went through that chubby stage when I was like between nine and ten. I was just constantly under scrutiny. (Marissa, 34, white)

> Yeah, I guess the point of that was my grandmother and the focus on obesity, like she is incredibly proud of my cousin who is like 120 [pounds] right now and she used to be my size. She made a point to show me these pictures before and after. It's really like prominent in her mind. She was also the one who wanted me to get my breasts reduced, whatever. She's like, "Why don't you do some plastic surgery? Why don't you do some plastic surgery?" I'm like, "I'm not doing plastic surgery." It's my body. If I'm going to do anything, it's not going to be on my boobs. [Laughs]. (Alice, 22, Latina)

Alice laughed as she was telling me about the interaction she had with her grandmother, but she was visibly annoyed and told me that her grandmother is fatphobic. Alice also told me that her culture—she's Brazilian—is the most "vain culture on the planet." She explained that plastic surgery is common in Brazil, and that a woman's appearance is more important than anything because women in Brazil try to meet the cultural expectations that Brazilian women are the most beautiful women in the world. Fat or chubby is not beautiful in Brazil—or in the United States.

In patriarchal societies, a woman's identity and self-esteem are grounded in her appearance and beauty (Wolf [1991] 2002). Parents and grandparents are sensitive to the fact that women are held to narrower standards of beauty, and they seem to recognize that discrimination in education and the workplace are likely for those who do not meet these rigid standards. They are also keenly aware that their daughters or granddaughters may have more difficulty attracting a suitable partner if she is "overweight" or "obese." In China, mothers broke and bound their daughter's feet to create an extremely small foot because the smaller the woman's foot, the better her chances at upward mobility. In Chinese culture, tiny feet were associated with fertility, beauty, and fidelity. Today, parents and grandparents encourage their daughters and granddaughters to exercise, watch what they eat, or diet if they are "too heavy" in order to improve their lot in life.

Tools to "Fix" the Abject Body
Dieting and Diet Culture

Research has shown that dieting behaviors among girls typically begin around 13 or 14 years of age and remain prevalent throughout adulthood (Huon and Lim 2000). Dieting is common among "normal" and "underweight" individuals, in addition to those who are "overweight" (Storz and Greene 1983). According to the Boston Medical Center website, approximately 45 million people are on a diet at any given time in the United States[4] and more than half the population has dieted at least once in their life. Scholars have identified three main types of dieting: (1) avoiding food consumption for long periods of time, (2) refraining from eating certain types of foods, and (3) restricting overall food consumption. All three diet types involve food restriction and an attempt to control one's appetite or eating behaviors mentally, rather than listening to one's body hunger or satiety cues (Higgins and Gray 1999).

Participants talked at length about how difficult it is to maintain caloric restriction. Most women said that it was impossible to live hungry all the time, and that as soon as they quit restricting their food intake they would begin to regain any weight they lost. Mandy (32, white) said, "Yeah, but then I let myself get relaxed after that and I gained the weight back so I was kind of... I wasn't too happy with myself for allowing myself to gain the weight back and not keeping up with it, but that's kind of been the story of my dieting life is that I'll be really gung-ho for a while and then it's like, 'ugh, I just don't want to do this anymore.'" The story of Mandy's dieting life is one where her weight cycles. She went on to say, "I have tried all kinds of methods, but right now I am really trying to just kind of, like, monitor how much I'm eating and I am focusing somewhat on what I'm eating." But she is not *just* watching what she eats; she is also injecting herself daily with a drug that is used to treat Type 2 diabetes—Victoza—which is helping curb her appetite: "I do not feel ravenous all the time or like I'm hungry all the time." Mandy does not have diabetes (and Victoza is not approved for weight loss), but Mandy and her husband have access to the drug because her father-in-law is an endocrinologist. Without Victoza, Mandy said she is hungry all the time and is unable to maintain caloric restriction. I asked her, "What happens when you stop taking it and your appetite comes back?" She replied that by then she will have trained her body to eat less and it will not be an issue. Victoza, in her mind, is a tool to train her body to require less food so that she can lose weight and maintain the weight loss.

Her body is an object separate from her *real self*—her controlled and thinner self. In the preceding anecdote, she said that she relaxed and "allowed" herself to gain the weight back, implying that she is not disciplined enough to ignore her corporeal demands. Among these women, it was common for them to discuss weight gain in this manner. They talked about how they "failed" to keep the weight off or "got lazy" and quit restricting what they ate daily. They seemed to view their fat selves similarly to how the larger culture views fat persons—as lazy, undisciplined, out of control, and gluttonous—but when they lost weight, they felt that they had "tamed" their body and were in control. For the most part, they were convinced that they could maintain the weight loss if they worked hard and did not "get lazy" again. They had internalized the messages that are purported by the larger culture about fat persons and worked hard to "prove" that they possessed the willpower to "train their body" to eat less.

In the following quote, Nicole (25, white) reveals that she feels like a failure because she gained back the weight she had lost previously. The language she uses is similar to Mandy's in that she accepts blame for her body size: "I feel like even if I think that I'm a failure in terms of my weight, I'm clearly not a failure in terms of my education. I feel like having a Master's and going for my PhD and being able to show that I'm a very smart person makes it easier for me to not feel like everybody thinks I'm a fuck-up because I couldn't keep the weight off. Because I know everybody thought it, but yet, how could they not?" In addition to failing to control her weight, she dissociates from herself, too. She wants people to know that she is smart and not a "complete" failure. By discussing her education, she is also attempting to show others that she has willpower. She might not be able to maintain control over her body, but she is disciplined enough to complete a master's degree and is making progress toward a PhD.

Weight loss through diet alone is extraordinarily difficult to maintain, and most people who lose weight will regain the weight they lost within one year (Field et al. 2003), which is yet another paradox of dieting. Those who dieted the most, at least in this sample, were typically the largest. Yet diets are exceptionally popular in US culture. According to an ABC news article,[5] the diet industry rakes in approximately $20 billion from diet books, diet drugs, and weight-loss surgeries, and 108 million people are dieting in the United States at any given point in time. According to Marketdata Enterprises, in 2013 the diet industry will reach $66 billion, which they attribute to weight gain that took place during the recession.[6]

Despite the fact that there is so much pressure to diet or to maintain a "thin" body, there is also tremendous pressure to engage in social eating and to "splurge" at parties. This is the paradox of the diet culture. Numerous women talked about how difficult it is to stick to a diet when in the presence of other people, especially at parties or during the holidays because (1) there is not food available that is "healthy" or (2) others are "breaking the dieting rules," and those who are "breaking the rules" want everyone else to do the same so that they do not feel guilty for indulging:

> I'm diabetic now and I'm trying to lose weight. I'm at 289. My highest weight was 307. I've been slowly and steadily, healthfully trying to change the way I eat and my relationship with food. This potluck, everybody knowing I'm diabetic and I'm not the only one, there's two of us in the office of eight that are diabetic, one who had a stroke a year and a half ago, so he shouldn't be eating that way either, but it'll be a potluck, and I'm expected to participate. I'll bring the salad and everybody else brings donuts, pastries, and four different kinds of cakes. There's one thing I can eat in the entire place, and then the rest is just garbage food. (Linda, 40, white)

Linda is frustrated because the diet culture and her medical condition have rendered her hyper(in)visible. Diet culture—or capitalism in general—demands that we purchase products to help us lose weight so that we will overconsume products that might lead to weight gain; this is one the paradoxes of dieting (Hesse-Biber 2007). Diet culture operates by dictating that people avoid eating sugar or foods high in fat or carbohydrates most of the time, but if they have "been good" and stuck to their diet, then they deserve to "splurge" on occasion. Parties are the perfect excuse to "cheat" on their diet or "reward" themselves for sticking so closely to their diet for a variety of reasons: (1) parties are relatively infrequent and are not daily occurrences; (2) people are *supposed* to relax during a celebration and not worry about indulging; and (3) parties frequently feature foods that are forbidden on the diet because they contain high quantities of fat, sugar, or carbohydrates. When one consumes these "bad foods," they often frame it as "being bad" because they are not sticking to their diet.

Linda is hyper(in)visible because her diabetes prevents her from joining her coworkers in the indulgences of the party. Other women I spoke with, who did not have diabetes but were dieting, reported feeling similarly about not being able to indulge with everyone else. Many said that they were actually harassed by family members or friends about not eating cake, cookies, or other foods that were "forbidden" on their diet. It is paradoxical because these are the same family members who had pressured them to diet in the first place; a common sentiment was that no matter what they do, they are doing something wrong.

Numerous women talked about work-related diets, meaning that coworkers decide collectively to "all go on a diet" or their place of employment contracts with a diet program as part of an employee wellness program. Typically, the program required some additional payment from the employee, and the meetings or other activities were held at the end of the workday.[7] In both of these situations—potlucks or work-sponsored diets—food and eating habits become highly visible, especially for women whose bodies are large. What they are eating or not eating, whether they have joined the weight-loss group, what they bring to the potluck, or whether they engage in "fat talk" can influence how they are treated at work.

Fernanda, a 36-year-old Latina schoolteacher, told me about the diet program that her school has adopted. She said that she has not joined the group because she felt like it would trigger unhealthy eating habits (i.e., too much restriction). She reportedly has been working hard to eat healthfully (she defined it as limiting processed foods and avoiding animal products) rather than restrict, because she has had a tendency to become obsessive and gain more weight in the end. However, she feels like she is missing important face time with the principal and vice principal because she has not joined the diet group and they have. She also thinks that people at work question why she has not joined, especially because she is one of the larger teachers at her school. The diet culture at work has made her both hypervisible because she is not participating and hyperinvisible when it comes to face time with her supervisors. The fact that she has not joined the group also pushes her to the margins of hyper(in)visibility because of the assumption that fat individuals have a responsibility to lose weight. If she does not join the group then she is irresponsible, lazy, or deviant, and of course, these are not characteristics one wants to project at work.

Dieting is often combined with exercise as a weight-loss tool, and the majority of the women I spoke with regularly engage in exercise. For some, exercise is used in addition to caloric restriction for weight loss; for others, it is used in lieu of caloric restriction. For a small group of women I interviewed, exercise had nothing to do with weight loss or weight maintenance; it was instead discussed as a way to relieve stress or for health. Participants explained that exercise presents some interesting challenges, especially for those at the heavier end of the weight spectrum.

One young woman recounted a story about a gym owner in her hometown who was petrified that the equipment would not support her weight. Another woman told me that even though she has been going to the same gym for years, the staff, especially new hires, frequently became concerned about her because her face gets really red when she is working out. She said they approach her and ask if she is OK. She assumed that they thought she was going to pass out or have a heart attack because she was fat and presumably "out of shape."

With the exception of exercise that takes place in the home, most people exercise in public, which makes fat persons who exercise highly visible. Numerous women reported having other gym customers stare at them. One woman even told me that a young (thin) woman said to her, "It's people like you who make the rest of us look bad." Fortunately, a trainer at the gym overheard the comment and asked the young woman to leave, but the fact that fat women are bullied at the gym makes many reluctant to go in the first place. Due to the high visibility of such activities, some women also complained about the fact that they could not find adequate workout clothes, such as sports bras, in their size. Not having "proper" attire for the gym not only prevented some women from engaging in exercise but made others who did so stand out even more because they were not dressed "appropriately." One woman told me that she buys the largest size available and that is still too tight. But she wears it anyway so that she can attend her yoga class.

Dieting remains popular among women and many men despite the finding that dieting to control weight is often times ineffective. Unfortunately, researchers have also found that dieting can sometimes lead to disordered eating behaviors or a preoccupation with food and body size (Neumark-Sztainer et al. 2006).

Disordered Eating Behaviors

Eating disorders are classified as psychological disorders in the *Diagnostic Statistical Manual of Mental Disorders* (DSM-V; American Psychiatric Association 2013), and they are differentiated as anorexia nervosa, bulimia nervosa, binge eating disorder (BED), and eating disorders not otherwise specified (EDNOS). It is estimated that 10 million people in the United States suffer from eating disorders such as anorexia and bulimia, and if binge eating disorder is included, millions more are afflicted. However, these estimates are fairly conservative due to the strictness of the criteria employed, limited access to a physician or mental-health professional trained to diagnosis the disorder, and underdiagnosis for groups such as men and racial/ethnic minorities.[8]

EDNOS, or disordered eating, includes severe caloric restriction, compulsive exercise, bingeing, purging, and the elimination of specific foods (i.e., avoiding fats or carbohydrates). Increasingly, EDNOS is recognized as similar to anorexia or bulimia with regard to its negative health consequences. Health risks associated with disordered eating include cardiovascular problems, amenorrhea, renal complications, blood dysfunction, hypothermia, and osteoporosis (American Psychiatric Association 2013). According to Cogan (1999, 232), despite the prevalence and health risks, EDNOS is not included in the typical training for physicians and dieticians and is largely ignored as a public health issue.

Eating disorders and disordered eating have often been assumed to affect white, young, privileged women, yet the "new recruits" include men, children under ten, racial and ethnic minorities, and women in mid and late life (Hesse-Biber 2007). In essence, eating disorders are affecting a larger number of people, yet some groups such as fat women are ignored. In popular culture, thin young women who engage in disordered eating practices are often viewed as victims of society's preoccupation with thinness (Saguy and Gruys 2010), and eating disorders are frequently glamorized and associated with discipline and control. In other words, someone who appears emaciated is thought to have tremendous willpower, whereas someone who is "obese" is assumed to lack discipline and control. Because bodies that are "too thin" are celebrated and bodies that are "too fat" are abhorred, it becomes unimaginable to most, even well-educated folks, that a fat person is starving herself. Therefore, many fat women who starve themselves or binge and purge are ignored and overlooked—they are hyper(in)visible.

Some of the women I spoke with discussed their eating and/or exercise behaviors as disordered, but many did not, and while it is not my intention to diagnose or pass judgment, some of their eating behaviors met the DSM-V guidelines for disordered eating, especially EDNOS and binge eating disorder (Field et al. 2003; Patton et al. 1999). For example, consider the following two narratives:

> I'm under 1,000 calories a day now. My lunch is my big meal, then I will have a piece of fruit in the afternoon, and then I have a protein bar for dinner. That seems to be helping me get back on track and making food less important. That's been a huge a thing for me, is making food less important and more about having nutrition versus social—I don't go out and eat all the time with my friends anymore. (Katrina, 31, white)

> Periodically, I would put myself through whatever I had to in order to lose enough weight in order to be acceptable . . . and I think that took more of a toll on me emotionally than anything else. (Marilyn, 60, white)

Both Katrina and Marilyn talked about fairly severe caloric restriction for weight loss. In Katrina's case, less than 1,000 calories a day is considered too few to allow for proper bodily function, especially for someone who is as active as Katrina. She is a belly dancer and aerobics class instructor, so she said she typically exercises for approximately two hours per day. Katrina's need to keep her caloric intake at 1,000 calories a day has isolated her from her friends and made her invisible. Marilyn did not specify how many calories she typically consumes, but she described many of her diets as "crash diets"; she said she severely restricted her food intake by skipping meals and drinking meal replacement shakes.

Some of the women I interviewed reportedly suffered health consequences as a result of extreme dieting, but in Carol's case, the adults in her life did not recognize the behavior as problematic or dangerous:

> It was disordered. I was really, really stringent on what I would eat. I didn't eat much at all. I wasn't as bad as I was when I was in eighth grade; I went on a huge crash diet. I only ate 800 calories a day, and I lost 100 pounds as well, which I think is really incredible for a kid that age, but my hair started coming out. I started blacking out. My periods stopped. So I knew that I had to start eating again, and I could—the weight was just flying back on that point, and that's just such a hard age to begin with, like I had lost 100 pounds. I was down to 180 pounds. But tell me when 180 was good. So teachers would say, "Oh, you're doing such a fantastic job, keep it up." But to all the other kids, I was still fat ass. (Carol, 30, white)

Carol was still a "fat ass" to the kids because she was still much larger than the average teenager, but the fact that her periods stopped and her hair started falling out indicates that her severe caloric restriction was taking a toll on her body. Note that her teachers encouraged her to "keep up the good work," despite the fact that it was having disastrous consequences on her health. Lupe (33, Latina) told me that she was hospitalized for an eating disorder in her late teens; she lost enough weight that she was considered emaciated and met the criteria for anorexia nervosa: "I was not eating, and when I ate I would throw everything up. I was exercising three hours a day and then eventually I did go to the hospital because I was very—I got very sick and everything." Lupe is the only woman I interviewed who told me that she had been diagnosed with anorexia nervosa, but plenty of other women met the criteria for bulimia nervosa and EDNOS.

The majority of the women I spoke with who either purged or severely restricted never got to the point where anyone would "recognize" that they had an eating disorder, even if they had physical problems as a result of their behavior. In fact, most received praise for their weight-loss efforts, as Carol indicated. If one does not become emaciated or "thin enough," the fact that her behaviors are harmful or dangerous is often ignored, rendered invisible, and typically overlooked. Moreover, some of the participants were prescribed "extreme diets" from their physicians. Beth (60, white) describes one of many physician-monitored diets that she has tried over the years: "I went on the hCG diet, another physician supervised diet. hCG is supposed to break down your fat, put it in your system, and then it goes out, but really what it is, is eating 500 calories a day—so less than a concentration camp diet. And there I lost a hundred pounds really, really fast, but then I was so sick. I was 20 and when I came off that diet I was so sick, and I had the first abnormal pap smear I'd ever had, and I've been having them ever since." Whether Beth's severe restriction caused her abnormal pap smear is not clear, but she was not well and she believes that the extreme diet has had lasting physical consequences.

Some physicians prescribe Very Low Calorie Diets (VLCD), even though many health-care professionals consider it disordered and dangerous. Berg (1999) reviewed the research on VLCD and found that these diets carry severe health risks, even when medically monitored, and that they are generally ineffective. Yet despite the risks and poor results, VLCD are frequently still recommended for patients with a BMI greater than 30 or for those with a BMI of 27 to 30 who have a comorbid condition. The stated rationale is that fat people need to lose weight quickly to reduce their risk factors, even though a safe and conservative treatment may be more appropriate.

One of the problems with excessive caloric restriction is binging. When one denies their body food, the body goes into a starvation mode where it expends fewer calories while waiting for food to become plentiful again. And when the body is in this mode, people crave fat and sugar because these are the substances that are best suited to help the body deal with caloric scarcity. Some researchers argue that this can create a cycle of binging and restriction, which can impact metabolism as well. During the binge episode, the body, afraid it will starve again, stores the food as fat, which could be why countless dieters end up gaining more weight than they lost (Miller 1999). Nicole (25, white) said, "Before the Atkins diet, I spent a lot of time in middle school doing Slim Fast, and through high school. I would drink those and take the bars to school and stuff, but that didn't really work because I would be really hungry and I'd eat a lot when I got home." As Nicole says, severe restriction does not typically work because dieters are so hungry that when they are presented with the opportunity to eat they frequently overeat. This theme was repeated with extraordinary frequency among this sample of women.

Some of the women I talked with had been diagnosed with binge eating disorder (BED), which is characterized by recurrent episodes of binge eating without the presence of inappropriate compensatory behaviors, including fasting, compulsive exercise, or purging, and involves both a subjective (loss of control) and objective (amount of food consumed) component (Stunkard and Allison 2003). Wendy has not been officially diagnosed with BED, but she thinks she has it, and she said that as long as she is not too stressed she can usually keep it under control:

> The official definition is pretty much what I do. I will indulge in greater quantities of food than most people would consider normal. Specific foods that are connected somehow to . . . it's not just emotional eating, but it is connected to my emotions. It feels like a compulsion. When it's triggered for me is when I'm in a situation where I'm under social pressure to eat a certain way. Then I feel like I have to go off by myself and have my food after, for instance, staying with family, family visits; that kind of thing. Being at a work-related conference, especially where I'm around a lot of women that I don't know well, because women do tend to judge each other on what we eat. (Wendy, 47, white)

Elaine, like Wendy, has not been officially diagnosed with BED, but Elaine said that her participation in Overeaters Anonymous (OA) taught her that she has a food addiction and BED. I asked her what made her think that, and she shared some of the behaviors that she had engaged in when she was compulsively eating:

> I mean normal people do not drive through a drive-thru and order for six people and then no matter what try to eat it without the

right utensils and get it all over themselves. Then trying to get in the house with it all over you to try to change clothes, you know what I mean. It was just a whole plethora of problems that was shrouded in secret eating that the awareness of it being so devastating to your health, your ego, your emotional health, that whole realm of this is wrong I need to try to find a way to fix it, to stop it, to treat it because it is so unhealthy. That was not there. The only awareness I had was what I had to do to fix the problem and to get the food ate and to get rid of it so that nobody would know. (Elaine, 52, white)

Both Wendy and Elaine discussed their behaviors as disordered. When Elaine was following the OA food plan she was able to lose some weight, but it did not last because she was not able to continue with the meetings. Elaine is suffering from numerous health problems, some related to her weight and some not. She is currently undergoing treatment for hepatitis C and is trying to lose weight. When we spoke, she was 441 pounds and needed to lose around 50 pounds so that she could be eligible for weight-loss surgery. Neither Wendy nor Elaine attribute their size directly to binging, but both know that it has had an impact, but it is not clear which came first.

For many of the women I spoke with, dieting seemed to precede binging behaviors, which is consistent with the literature. Reas and Grilo (2007) examined a group of clinically "overweight" adults diagnosed with BED. They were interested in the timing and sequence of the onset of "overweight," BED, and dieting. Findings indicated that the majority of the sample was not "overweight" because of binge eating: 63 percent of their sample was "overweight" prior to dieting and 21 percent dieted before they became "overweight" or engaged in BED. The results were congruent with earlier studies that found that "excess" weight and dieting typically precede BED (Field et al. 2003; Yanovski 2003).

The social construction of "obesity" and eating disorders are problematic because the emphasis is on a number (typically one's BMI), rather than health. Moreover, the focus is on individuals' behavior rather than social structures that contribute to disordered eating behaviors. Eating disorders are often assumed to affect young, relatively affluent women, and while there is great concern for those who are diagnosed with eating disorders, there is less attention paid to the millions of people who engage in harmful behaviors that are not diagnosed as disorders because they do not meet, or appear to meet, the extant criteria. More often than not, fat women are rendered hyper(in)visible when it comes to a diagnosis of an eating disorder (except BED), even though their behaviors are sometimes as equally destructive, and they may even be "prescribed an eating disorder." The extreme diets engaged in by the clear majority of the women in this study were unsuccessful, and many weigh more today than they did when they began trying to "fix" their bodies. For some, like Elaine, weight-loss surgery is their last hope at losing a significant amount of weight.

Weight-Loss Surgery

Of the 74 women I spoke with, 13 had weight-loss surgery (WLS), and 3 were hoping to have WLS in the future. There are several types of procedures, and they vary in effectiveness, side effects, and invasiveness. The least invasive procedure is gastric banding, also known as lap band or a sleeve. In this procedure, an inflatable band is inserted to squeeze the stomach into two sections: a smaller upper pouch and a larger lower section. The two sections are still connected, but the channel between them is very small, which slows down the emptying of the upper pouch. Gastric banding physically restricts the amount of food one can consume in a sitting. A slightly more invasive procedure is sleeve gastrectomy, which involves removing about 75 percent of the stomach. What remains of the stomach is a narrow tube or sleeve, which connects to the intestines. Finally, the most invasive procedure (and the most common) is gastric bypass or Roux-en-Y gastric bypass. A surgeon divides the stomach into two parts, which seals off the upper section from the lower. The surgeon then connects the upper stomach directly to the lower section of the small intestine. Essentially, the surgeon creates a shortcut for the food, bypassing a section of the stomach and the small intestine. Skipping these parts of the digestive tract means that fewer calories are absorbed.[9]

The women who had WLS had mixed feelings about the success of the procedure as well as the side effects. The most common side effects of gastric banding were the band slipping or vomiting due to overeating. Only one woman I talked with had sleeve gastrectomy, and she has had to have two follow-up procedures due to problems. Most of the women had Roux-en-Y gastric bypass and the side effects they reported were pretty similar, but the way that the women viewed the side effects differed fairly dramatically. For instance, Nancy related,

> *Nancy:* I couldn't lose weight. I was still in that mind-set that all of my problems will disappear if I'm suddenly skinny. And I started looking into gastric bypass surgery. And I ended up having the surgery five years ago, and had severe complications, including malnutrition, afterwards, combined with not being able to keep the weight off.
> *JG:* What sort of complications did you have, other than the malnutrition and . . .
> *Nancy:* Well, I lost all my hair. Luckily it has come back, but that was really traumatic. I have a tremendous amount of scar tissue in my abdomen. And so I have a lot of pain and pressure from that. B12 deficiency, which is leading to, unfortunately, neuropathy. Constant fatigue and depression issues because of it. So you know, it's coming to the realization that I'm actually probably going to live five to ten years less than what I would have if I wouldn't have had the surgery, and it's been quite a difficult thing. (Nancy, 35, white)

Nancy has suffered what she considers to be traumatic side effects and regrets her decision to have the surgery, especially because she has gained back the weight. However, others with similar problems see it as the price one pays to rid their bodies of the abject fat. Jasmine, who is slightly ambivalent about having had WLS, talked about another common side effect of gastric bypass surgery:

> *Jasmine:* The sugar thing—I can't do sugar at all because I get that dumping syndrome. That really turned out to be good for me because I was a sugaraholic or whatever you want to call it because I loved to eat candy, sweets, and stuff like that. I can't do that, so that's been great.
> *JG:* Can you explain dumping syndrome?
> *Jasmine:* That's where you get, just all of the sudden you get really sweaty, and you have to run to the bathroom because it's like you have diarrhea right away. It's just liquid that dumps. You just dump everything. It's really uncomfortable. On the other

hand, I could get real sweaty and I'll be vomiting just instantly after I eat. I can just get a sweet taste in my mouth and that can set it off. (Jasmine, 52, African American)

Jasmine did not have too many issues with her weight, but she has an illness that was exacerbated by the extra weight she was carrying around and felt that the only way she was going to be able to continue to work and live her life was to have the surgery. In fact, Jasmine told me that she was really uncomfortable with all the attention that she was getting as a result of the weight she has lost (93 pounds when we spoke). She said that she was so accustomed to not being seen, and that now she is really self-conscious, especially with the male gaze. She said that she is feeling better physically with the weight loss, and she does not regret having the surgery, but she said she was more confident and comfortable when she was larger. However, I spoke to others who expressed complete satisfaction with their decision to have weight-loss surgery, too: "Honestly it's the first time in my life I don't diet anymore. Most people go, 'Oh, it's so restrictive.' But it's not, it's actually really freeing because I eat small amounts. I eat healthy. I only have room for so much. I can't binge. I eat simple. It's been very freeing. I don't think about food. I know I eat protein first. It's become routine, it took all that mental energy that you put into dieting and whatnot away, and so it's been wonderful. Everybody goes, 'Oh, it's so restrictive.' But no, it's so freeing" (Barbara, 45, white).

Barbara, still technically considered "obese," has lost 290 pounds and is thrilled. She said that she feels free again. She had been at a point where she had lost mobility and was having a difficult time leaving the house and taking care of her son, but since the surgery, she said that she now goes hiking and swimming. Barbara told me that she was around 500 or so pounds because she suffered from BED. She knew that she had a problem and sought help from a counselor before her surgery, because "I knew that surgery would only help with the weight loss and that it would not fix my mind." Barbara is "free" from dieting and thinking about food because of gastric bypass surgery, but other women who talked with me "freed" themselves of the shackles of dieting through electing to stop dieting.

Calling It Quits

The popular culture and medical messages that we are inundated with focus on how important it is to lose weight or expel the fat from our bodies. So in that respect, the abject (fat) body is subversive because it resists discipline. Such a body defies normativity in its appearance, practice, and stylization and fails to situate itself easily in dominant categories and roles (Foucault 1977). Because the body is a site of investment, control, and cultural production, anomalous (abject or grotesque) bodies can be understood as threatening to the social order. The grotesque operates through juxtaposition and irony. Its primary feature is that its borders are ambiguous, and this ambiguity is not avoided—it's celebrated. A grotesque body can represent a refusal of orderliness and social control (Pitts 2003). Grosz (1990, 40) states that anorexia is a form of protest at the social meaning of the female body. Rather than seeing it simply as out-of-control compliance with the current patriarchal ideals of slenderness, it is precisely a renunciation of these "ideals."

I argue that this same claim could be made about fat women's bodies. Women who are fat also deny the patriarchal ideals of the "perfect" form because their bodies are often viewed as simultaneously masculine and feminine. It is particularly subversive when fat women reject the societal demands that they diet in an attempt to achieve the "ideal" female form. They resist discipline and social control, but it is not easy, as Brooke (35, white) discusses:

> There was a time that I really worked at it. I really worked to try to lose weight. I've gotten it—and then I'm sure you've heard that. I've done Weight Watchers, I've done . . . God, I can't even think of them all. I did meal plans. I've done the working out. I've done just smoking a pack of cigarettes a day without eating diet. I tried everything and I came to the point where I was like, in order for me to be a size 12 requires a constant sense of being hungry and control for the rest of my life and I don't want to do that anymore. If I can't do that anymore I've got to accept who I am. Because I can't, I just can't. Is it about willpower? No. I was kicked out at 18 and now I have a Master's degree all because I did it. That's not a person who lacks in willpower. I've come to this place where now I'm like, "You know what, I'm not going to try to obtain the

unobtainable." I've got to try to accept myself for who I am. That's tough. That's not easy.

Brooke's quote illustrates the frustration she has experienced over the years trying to lose weight. Some of the methods she has used are considered healthier than others, but none of them has led to lasting weight loss, and now she finds herself in the process of self-acceptance and learning to appreciate her body. The way she talks about this process demonstrates how incredibly difficult it is to overcome the idea that fat is abject. Marsha (58, white) expressed a similar sentiment about how challenging it is to lose weight:

> I would take some of it off. I did that when he [her son] was about four or five, I got not all the way as thin as I was before, but I got pretty far, way, way down again. But I did that working with a nutritionist and doing liquid protein breakfast and things like that. Which none of that's sustainable. In the last 10 or 15 years, the more I read and the more I study it and the more I understand is, every time you lose weight and regain it, it throws your metabolism off. It's gotten harder and harder to take it off. It's gotten impossible.

Marsha knows that she cannot stay on a strict diet for the rest of her life, and she also believes that the years of weight cycling have caused her metabolism to change. This was the conventional wisdom among this subsample of women. For the most part, this subset of women have educated themselves about dieting, weight loss, food, and metabolic processes, probably because they have spent a tremendous amount of time over the course of their lives trying to lose weight.

While many of the women reported that they have quit dieting and now focus on "healthful eating" and exercise, there was also evidence that they have not entirely accepted their bodies and would still like to lose weight: "I feel like I have done a lot of work over the years to accept myself physically. I ascribe to the HAES Philosophy, Health at Every Size®. I can still honestly tell you that if there was a pill with no side effects that I could take and I would be normal, I would do it" (Bonnie, 51, white). Bonnie has committed to healthful[10] eating and exercise, feels great physically, and no longer has high blood pressure or cholesterol, but she still wants to lose weight so that she is "normal." Nearly 80 percent of the sample reported engaging in regular exercise and are committed to eating healthy, whole foods. However, exercise and diet typically do not lead to drastic weight loss or at least the sort of weight loss that would put the majority of these women in the "normal" or even "overweight" BMI category. Those who do exercise and eat healthfully reported that they have lowered their diabetic risk, blood pressure, and cholesterol, even though the amount of weight they lost was insignificant.

Conclusion

In this chapter, I have illustrated how these women react to having a body that is abhorred and hyper(in)visible. I focused on three main issues: (1) how others have tried to control their bodies; (2) how they have employed a variety of tools in an attempt to expel their fat; and (3) how some have moved away from the dieting discourse and, despite the pressure, refrain from dieting. The women spoke about the stares they receive in public, the comments from strangers and loved ones about their bodies and food choices, and the tremendous pressure they feel to "fix" or change their body. The phenomenon of hyper(in)visibility functions as a mode of social control. In essence, the stares from strangers, the perceived pressure from loved ones, and the continual media attention on "obesity" communicated to these women that their bodies were not "normal" and that it was their responsibility to change it. The women discussed dieting, exercise, and weight-loss surgery as tools to expel the abject fat. The numerous ways these women have tried to lose weight led some to develop disordered eating behaviors, depression, anxiety, and fat hatred. Employing extreme methods to lose weight (i.e., disordered eating, bariatric surgery, or use of diet pills and amphetamines) has become normalized—even obligatory—for women who are fat.

In a society where fat is viewed as unattractive, disgusting, and irresponsible, it is not surprising that fat women begin to embody fat hatred and dissociate from their bodies. One need not look far to find a cornucopia of pills, plans, mixes, products, and procedures that are marketed for weight loss. Unfortunately, the majority of people do not have long-term success with diet pills or devices, and the dieter finds herself frequently feeling like a failure and moving on to another weight-loss tool. Of the current sample, 46 percent have quit dieting and decided that they are "no longer going to live a life where they are constantly seeking the newest weight-loss method." They have decided that they are not going to live their lives playing out a Sisyphean[11] struggle, forever trying and never succeeding. But it is extraordinarily difficult for most of these women to overcome the routines of secrecy and shame that they feel surrounding food, dieting, and their weight.

The few women in the sample who dieted themselves to a "normal" size at some point in their life described themselves as a fat person stuck in a thin person's body. They often felt that they were passing (Goffman 1963) as thin, that it was a façade and not their true identity, and that even though they did not want to gain weight, they felt more at home in their bodies when the weight returned.

As long as fat is considered a choice that can be changed through consumption of a product (i.e., diet products, surgery), we as a society will assume that fat people are responsible for the mistreatment they experience and leave unchallenged the view that fat is always unhealthy. By assuming that fat is an individual problem that can be changed through an individual's behaviors, we can easily ignore the social forces that have created a preoccupation with thinness and emphasis on one's appearance—and fat women will remain hyper(in)visible.

CHAPTER 4

FIT AND FAT

On June 18, 2013, the American Medical Association (AMA) voted to label "obesity" a disease, following a trend established earlier by the *International Classification of Diseases*, published by the World Health Organization.[1] Many who support the disease label argue that it will make treatment a priority and reduce stigma, because "obesity" will be recognized as a health problem rather than an individual failing. "The AMA's decision is an important step forward, and recognizes obesity as a serious and chronic condition that must be addressed as a priority for treatment in the medical field," said Rebecca Puhl, PhD, Rudd Center Director of Research and Weight Stigma Initiatives.[2] But others have major concerns.

Fat Studies scholars and activists are critical of the disease classification because now anyone with a body mass index (BMI) greater than or equal to 30, healthy or not, is automatically labeled as having a disease—"obesity." On one of the fat studies forums, members pointed out that a new priority to treat the disease "obesity" could render other ailments invisible, because "obesity" will now be the primary diagnosis. To be clear, this was already happening to many fat persons when they went to the doctor (Boero 2012), but now it is sanctioned.

For example, Claudialee, six years old and "obese," tragically died because she was misdiagnosed with Type 2 diabetes when she actually had Type 1 diabetes. Her doctor assumed she had Type 2 diabetes because she was fat, even though Type 2 diabetes is an adult disease and extremely rare in children under ten. The pediatrician told Claudialee's mother that Claudialee needed to lose weight. By the next appointment with the pediatrician, Claudialee had lost weight. Rather than recognizing the weight loss as a potential symptom of Type 1 diabetes (it is common for those with Type 1 diabetes to lose weight when the disease is not treated), the physician applauded Claudialee's mother and told her that the weight loss was evidence that the little girl's health was improving.

A couple months later, Claudialee died because her body shut down from the lack of insulin.[3] Claudialee died because she was fat and her fat made her disease, Type 1 diabetes, invisible because of the assumption that fat people have Type 2 diabetes. This is obviously an extremely tragic story, but it is not an isolated case, and some fear that this will become increasingly common because "obesity" itself is now labeled a disease—in essence, it has been fully medicalized.

Medicalization is the process by which medicine expands into areas that were not previously thought to be medical conditions such as alcoholism, drug abuse, and mental-health conditions like depression, anxiety, attention deficit disorder, and so forth. With medicalization, treatments are offered to "fix" a biomedical condition and remove blame from the individual. In other words, medicalization often works to remove the stigma associated with deviant behaviors such as alcoholism or drug abuse (Conrad and Schneider 1992). Yet with "obesity," despite the fact that it has been fully medicalized, the stigma is not waning. Conrad (1992, 223) distinguishes between medicalization and "healthicization" by stating that "medicalization proposes biomedical causes and interventions; healthicization proposes lifestyle and behavioral causes and interventions." Therefore, this slight distinction between the etiology and treatment of medicalized conditions like alcoholism and healthicized conditions like "obesity" perhaps explains why stigma reduction is unlikely with the disease labeling of "obesity."

As Hannele Harjunen (2009) points out, the medical discourse about fat is taken as the "truth" by medical professionals and the public alike. Fat has been treated as a health problem or medical concern for some time, but the recent move to officially label "obesity" a disease creates new challenges. Wann (2009) worries that the medicalization (or perhaps healthicization) of fat has led to increasing discrimination by health-care providers because of the assumption that fat can be treated or cured. The supposition is that if one is fat, despite all the available options to first prevent it or cure it, then the person who is fat must be lazy or unwilling to take care of him or herself.

Abigail Saguy (2013) found that people who read news reports where fat is discussed as a public health crisis are more likely to hold the opinion that fat is unhealthy and to express fatphobia. However, people who read news articles in which a point is made to demonstrate that one can be both fit and fat or that speak out against size discrimination are less likely to employ antifat attitudes or believe that fat represents a public health crisis. The way that the message is framed matters for the way the public views the issue. But it is not just the lay public who is affected by this framing.

Research indicates that physicians, nurses, and medical students believe that fat is preventable, that people who are fat are repulsive and overindulgent, that fat persons have family problems, that their fatness is the result of laziness, and that they are unsuccessful (Bagley et al. 1989; Blumberg and Mellis 1980; Hoppe and Ogden 1997; Klein et al. 1982; Maiman et al. 1979; Maroney and Golub 1992; Price et al. 1987). The women I interviewed frequently cited negative attitudes and mistreatment from physicians and other health-care providers as one of the reasons they avoid preventative care. With the new disease label, some fat activists fear that health-care providers will more frequently prescribe weight-loss medications and weight-loss surgery, both of which have histories of being unsafe and ineffective for long-term weight loss.[4]

Additional concerns by Fat Studies scholars and activists revolve around the fact that the new disease category could exacerbate the already tense relationship many fat persons have with physicians and other health-care professionals. Ragen Chastain, author of the blog *Dances with Fat*, offers advice for people who are fat as they prepare for a doctor's visit.[5] In the blog post "What to Say at the Doctor's Office," Ragen not only addresses some of the typical problems that fat persons encounter when seeing a physician but also provides postcards that one can take to the doctor's office as a reminder of what to say. For example, two important questions to ask the physician are "Do thin people get this health problem? What do you recommend for them?"

Ragen wrote the blog because she knows how difficult it is for many people who are fat to overcome "white coat anxiety," and she understands how important it is that fat patients be prepared to advocate for themselves. She wrote that she has been prescribed weight loss for a broken toe, a separated shoulder, and strep throat. Numerous women I interviewed revealed strikingly similar interactions with physicians. They had innumerable ailments attributed to their body size, such as sprained ankles, sore throats, sinus infections, acne, and so forth. Moreover, as I was talking about Fat Studies and the "obesity epidemic" in class, a student—who as she began to tell the story said, "Obviously I'm not a small girl"—volunteered that a doctor told her that she would suffer fewer colds if she lost weight. The class was horrified and wanted to know how a physician could be so ignorant. I explained that according to the women I interviewed and the numerous conversations I have been privy to in the "fat-o-sphere," this was unfortunately a common occurrence.

In the remainder of this chapter, I argue that the neoliberal focus on health (especially the assumption that thinness signifies health) and the medicalization or healthicization of fat perpetuates the hyper(in)visibility of fat women. To explain this process, the women's voices demonstrate the complex notions of what constitutes health in their eyes and how they have been treated within the health-care system. The phenomenon of hyper(in)visibility is perpetuated when physicians attribute any and all health ailments to participants' size (fat) while simultaneously rendering participants' knowledge of their own bodies and symptoms invisible. Hyper(in)visibility is further reinforced when equipment such as blood pressure cuffs, gowns, and other medical screening devices cannot physically accommodate the body of larger persons.

A substantial proportion of the women I interviewed discussed the Health at Every Size (HAES)® framework as an alternative to the hegemonic health paradigm (the view that fat is unhealthy and the only way to improve health is through weight loss). HAES® emphasizes size acceptance, taking care of one's body with enjoyable exercise and a nutritious varied diet, and listening to one's internal bodily cues (Bacon 2010; Burgard 2009).

Health as a Moral Obligation

As I discussed in Chapter 1, the Centers for Disease Control (CDC) frames "obesity" and being "overweight" as social problems (see also Kwan and Graves 2013) that put the "health" of the country at risk. Kwan and Graves (2013) note that embedded within this message is the idea that health is an intrinsic good and a metaphor for productivity, individual discipline, and purpose. In a neoliberal society, citizens are made to feel as though it is their moral duty to be healthy or that they should aim to be healthy (Rose 1999; Tischner and Malson 2012). This burden disproportionately affects women, because it is typically women who are responsible for maintaining their family's health through meal preparation, arranging doctor's visits, and ensuring that their children are physically active and well cared for (see also Boero 2012; Tischner 2013).

"Healthism," a concept coined by Robert Crawford (1980), is a preoccupation with health and well-being. It is grounded in the idea that health is something that anyone can achieve—if they work hard enough—and that it is one's individual and moral responsibility to maintain their health. The increasing emphasis in Western culture on being healthy or maintaining optimal health is not necessarily the result of individual choices. Disciplinary medicine relies on the illusion of personal choice (Murray 2008). But healthism or healthicization compels us to make choices that are in line with public health initiatives (see also Becker 1986; Kwan and Graves 2013). If we do not meet the public health prescription for optimal health (thinness), then we are (potentially) deemed morally inept and irresponsible (Conrad 1987). In essence, healthicization (surveillance medicine; Armstrong 1995) implores individuals to change their behaviors, and unlike medicalization, there is no absolution from moral judgment and accountability.

Furthermore, many argue that "obesity" threatens the economic health of society through billions of dollars in health-care costs and lost wages (Cawley and Meyerhoefer 2012; Trogdon et al. 2008). Again, this is part of the neoliberal requirement that citizens maintain their "health" so that they can work and participate in the economy (Foucault 1994). "Healthy" citizens are crucial to the modern neoliberal state because they keep it functioning with minimal economic burdens. Deborah Lupton (2012) argues that states sponsor programs that monitor and encourage weight loss, with the help of medical, public health, and social science experts who frame fat as a disease, to keep their citizenry controlled and more productive (see also Saguy 2013).

Moreover, neoliberal societies stress the importance of "freedom," "free choice," and individual responsibility. As part of the free market enterprise, consumers have abundant choices, but they are also expected to understand the risks associated with particular products and demonstrate the capacity for self-discipline. As I discussed in Chapters 1 and 3, the popular belief is that if people want to lose weight they should "push themselves away from the table and get off the couch" (numerous women told me that they could not even begin to count how many times they heard this exact phrase). The emphasis on individual responsibility for body weight and health status means that it is acceptable to blame individuals who are unhealthy or "obese" for their condition, because it is their fault for not behaving differently (see also Lupton 2012; Murray 2008; Saguy and Riley 2005). When health problems began to develop in some of the women I interviewed, they—not surprisingly—blamed their weight, even when it was unlikely that their condition was caused by their weight.

"Obesity" is framed as a pressing and potentially catastrophic social problem for North America and perhaps the entire world, as the term *globesity* reflects. In fact, the mainstream medical perspective that considers "obesity" a severe health risk is generally accepted as a commonsense truth (Campos 2004; Cogan and Ernsberger 1999). However, the emphasis on the harms of fat does not match the plethora of research that challenges the conventional wisdom that fat is always unhealthy. Studies have shown that extreme thinness is associated with increased mortality and that moderate "obesity" is associated with optimal health (Cao et al. 2014; Ernsberger and Haskew 1987; Garner and Wooley 1991). Others have found that poor health outcomes among the "obese" may be related to histories of weight cycling, health consequences associated with discrimination and stigma, and the fact that many fat persons tend to avoid physicians and preventive care for fear that they will be chastised for their weight (Ernsberger 2009; Lyons 2009). Despite the counterevidence, it appears to be incredibly difficult for most people to believe that someone who is fat could possibly be healthy.

Visibly Unhealthy

In contemporary society, fat symbolizes unhealthiness, which makes it difficult for most people—including physicians—to see beyond the fat and recognize that some ailments might not be related to adiposity. Participants understandably became angry when their sore throats or headaches were attributed to their weight, but they also were often uncritically willing to accept that many other conditions they experienced were related to their weight—even when they knew they had a genetic predisposition or that there was no evidence that the condition was weight related. Given the cultural emphasis on healthism and the individual responsibility associated with healthiness, it is not surprising that most of the women blamed themselves (or their fat) for their health problems. Meredith relays this mind-set here:

> I started having health issues; I had high blood pressure for a long time, which was not very unusual because it runs in both sides of my family—maternal and paternal. But then I had some issues where I started having heart palpitations, that kind of thing, then I had to have a breast biopsy and I was too large to have the needle biopsy so they had to do surgery to have it done. And at that point I was talking with my primary physician and he's like, "Have you really considered the [gastric bypass] surgery?" And I'm like, I said "Yes and no" and he's like, "Why not?" and I said, "Because I have seen what can happen, that was bad." And he talked to me quite some time about it and he was right. I only see the bad things that happened, I don't—you don't get to see the good part of what happens after people—somebody who has the surgery and they do great and you don't ever see them again. (Meredith, 52, white)

Meredith did not have breast cancer, and her high blood pressure was likely inherited, but she attributed these health conditions to her weight and proceeded to have gastric bypass surgery. When we met, Meredith was nine months postsurgery and had lost one hundred pounds, but she was still "obese" and was hoping to lose more weight to "improve her health." Meredith knows many conditions are genetic (she is a registered nurse), but she made it quite clear that she thought that most people's health problems (hers included) were the result of lifestyle decisions, such as not eating right or not exercising enough. She uncritically accepted the view that fat is unhealthy and the source of numerous health problems.

Meredith wanted me to know that her daughter was not going to "make the same mistake I did," and she exercises twice a day and strictly monitors her diet and her daughter's diet. She told me a story to demonstrate the importance of instilling healthy food choices in her granddaughter. The three of them (Meredith, her daughter, and granddaughter) were at the zoo and they took a break so her granddaughter could have a snack (orange slices). She said that sitting next to them was another family with a toddler, about the same age as her granddaughter, and that they were giving her ice cream. She expressed disappointment that the other family was feeding their toddler ice cream, because she sees individual behaviors such as eating ice cream as tied to the "obesity" problem. Meredith told me about this event because to her it provided visual "evidence" that parents are not teaching their children how to eat healthfully.

For many in the Western world, visually observing that someone is fat serves as "knowledge" that the fat person is unhealthy (Burgard 2009; Murray 2008). This theme was echoed in quite a few of the statements made by participants as we discussed health generally and their own health more specifically: "Well, I don't think it's about being skinny. I think it's about being your best, being at your best health-wise, you know, and you can—certainly, just because you're skinny, doesn't mean you're healthy but for sure, if you're fat, you're not healthy" (Aisha, 31, African). Aisha makes it clear that she does not believe it is possible for a fat person to be healthy. Fat itself is evidence of ill health. It was common for the women I talked with to slip back and forth between discussing health and weight loss, because many of them saw weight loss as a key component necessary to improve their health. Sally said, "And so, then I've got to work on trying to lose weight on top of having a thyroid condition; that is always a battle. What I've learned is that if you're not active you can't even begin to lose weight. So, I'm doing it—I just decided that I had to become healthy"

(Sally, 46, white). Sally has hypothyroidism (underactive thyroid), which was not caused by her weight but can lead to weight gain if left untreated.

According to the Mayo Clinic, hypothyroidism is caused by a number of factors, such as iodine deficiency, autoimmune disorders, medications, pregnancy, and so forth. Sally knows that a side effect of hypothyroidism is weight gain—because an underactive thyroid slows metabolism—so she has to "work hard" to lose weight or at least not gain more weight. Her statement that she "has to become healthy" indicates that she views health as directly related to body weight.

Tracey also wants to lose weight, but she was quick to let me know that her reasons for weight loss are not wrapped up in appearance. She told me that her desire to lose weight is purely about health:

> Then the issue for me is not that I think that I'm ugly, or that I think fat is ugly. I don't at all. It's that I want to be healthier. I want to live forever. Because I know statistically, people who are as fat as I am don't live as long as people who are at a healthy weight, and I don't want to be one of those people. I don't want to die young. There is so much more that I could do. I get out of breath pretty easily, just from doing regular household stuff or even [low voice] even like standing in front of a room full of people and presenting, I have to really modulate and regulate my breath so I don't get out of breath just from standing around. (Tracey, 32, white)

Tracey noted that the only "health problem" she currently has is that she easily gets out of breath. But she is nonetheless worried that she is going to die young from being fat. Fat does not necessarily cause shortness of breath, but low cardiovascular fitness does. In other words, thin people who smoke or have low levels of cardiovascular fitness also become winded quite easily, but instead of recognizing that she might need to focus on her cardiovascular fitness, she focuses entirely on her weight as the problem. In this manner, physical ailments are reduced to body weight rather than lifestyle or activities.

Fernanda, a 36-year-old Latina, said that one of the main reasons she agreed to the interview was because she wanted to talk about her experiences with medical professionals when she was pregnant. She told me that during one of the first meetings with her midwife she became incredibly scared because the midwife expressed concern about her weight and warned her of the dangers of being fat and pregnant. The midwife assumed that Fernanda had health problems because of her weight—Fernanda did not and still does not have any health problems. I asked her, "Did you tell her that you are healthy?" She responded, "It felt like, 'How can I say that I'm healthy if I have extra pounds? How can I say . . .' It's like, 'Obviously you're not,' that kind of thing." Fernanda did not believe she could be healthy because her body size provided "evidence" that she was not.

Fernanda is a vegetarian and prepares nearly all her family meals from scratch because she is worried about preservatives and additives. She is also quite active. She has a toddler, attends a Bikram yoga class several times per week, and is an elementary school teacher. However, despite her healthful eating, regular exercise, and lack of health problems, she believes that she is not healthy. It became clear to me as Fernanda and I talked that it was not just about her health; it was also about her appearance, as it was for numerous others I spoke to. Fernanda told me,

> I worry that I will develop some diseases or something that they talk about, like diabetes or . . . I don't have any of that stuff, but I worry that I may get it. Now my thinking is maybe I need to cut out milk and eggs and stuff, because we basically are vegetarian, but we have milk and eggs. Then maybe it's that, maybe that's what I need to cut out. How could I get to where I wouldn't be overweight? I would like to really kind of turn . . . make sure that my health . . . I think that it's good now, but I'd like to make sure that going forward it would be really good, especially with children or with a two-year-old. It's like, "Oh my gosh, I need to be." I feel like my mental state will be clearer and stuff like that. (Fernanda, 36, Latina)

Fernanda does not have any health problems, but she is worried. What was so interesting about this portion of the interview is that I had asked her about her health. Yet she nearly immediately went on to discuss weight loss. This was a common occurrence among the women I talked with. They, like the rest of the culture, seemed to be unable to separate health from body size. Fernanda even thinks that losing weight might make her a better mom because she thinks her mind is clouded from her weight. I asked her if she was experiencing difficulty concentrating and she said no. Again, weight is to blame for everything—even things that are not a problem.

Paige, who is concerned that she might end up alone like her fat aunt, was convinced not only that is it impossible to be healthy and fat but also that being fat was keeping her from engaging in "normal activities":

> But maybe technically you're not *unhealthy* on paper as a person could be who is at your size or anyone could be. It's tough though, when you see yourself not living up to what you could be, you don't want to overestimate how healthy you are. Because you're like, well, I couldn't even jog for five minutes straight, how healthy could I be? I feel I got lucky that I'm not more unhealthy than I am, at the same time, I don't want to say . . . I have a thyroid condition, I have reflux, and I potentially have PCOS and I'm not physically capable of some things that the average person should probably be physically capable of doing, if they were healthy. (Paige, 28, white)

I asked her what things, and she said things like "being able to run to catch a bus, fitting comfortably on the seat in the bus, playing tennis, those sorts of things." When we spoke, she was playing tennis every Saturday with her father and working out four or five days a week. She had lost a little weight, nothing substantial, but noted her cardiovascular fitness was greatly improved and that she had more energy.

Paige's hypothyroidism has likely contributed to her weight gain (or difficulty losing weight), as has polycystic ovarian syndrome (PCOS). PCOS is an endocrine disorder characterized by weight gain, irregular menstruation, acne, infertility, and male pattern hair growth and loss (Fisancik 2009, 106). Of the women I spoke with, 13 had been diagnosed with PCOS. For some, they started to gain weight extremely rapidly like Rochelle, the woman I discussed in Chapters 1 and 2, but for others the diagnosis came after years of having physicians blame acne and irregular periods on the woman's "obesity." In fact, several were told that if they lost weight their acne would disappear and their periods would regulate—in this manner their actual health conditions were rendered hyperinvisible because of their body size. None of Paige's health problems were caused by her weight. In fact, quite the opposite is likely the case, because two of her conditions cause weight gain. Yet she attributes her "poor health" to her weight and as evidence that being fat is unhealthy.

Fat frequently serves as a scapegoat for any and all medical conditions. If one is fat and one has a health problem, then fat is to blame, or in Murray's (2008, 80) words, "Fat flesh always already confesses a pathology, by virtue of its very visible difference." The hypervisible fat body is evidence of a disease, and when an actual physical ailment is present, fat is the cause. Barbara, 45 and white, echoed this thinking when she said, "Then I had uterine cancer, again due to my weight, so my son's adopted." I asked Barbara why she thought the uterine cancer was caused by her weight, and she told me that the doctors told her that fat women produce more estrogen than thin women and uterine cancer is caused by excess estrogen production. It is important to note that thin women also develop uterine cancer, so one cannot establish a causal link between fat and uterine cancer.

According to numerous "obesity" researchers, gynecological cancers are more prevalent and more deadly among fat women than thin women (Amy et al. 2006). However, the question remains whether fat causes gynecological cancer or whether fat women are less likely to be diagnosed early because they avoid routine exams. According to Amy and colleagues, women with BMIs above 30 delayed cancer-screening tests and thought that their body size prevented them from receiving quality health care. Countless women that I interviewed indicated that they avoid going to the doctor at all costs, especially gynecologists, even though they have health insurance and know that they should not avoid preventative care.

Just as many diseases and ailments are readily attributed to a person's fat, there are also diseases that are almost entirely ignored. Lipedema, a seriously understudied and underdiagnosed ailment, affected two of the women I spoke with.[6] Lipedema is characterized by symmetrical swelling of the lower body—namely, the legs and hips, but not the feet. As Wendy discusses, it often begins to manifest during puberty, and in 90 percent of cases there is a hormonal disruption (pituitary, thyroid, or ovarian): "I have, as it turns out, a hereditary condition called lipedema, which causes the lower body to . . . it affects the way the lower body stores fat. It causes a specific fat appearance in the hips, thighs, and legs. You can look this up, but it says it almost universally occurs in women. It sets in at puberty. It becomes worse at pregnancy—which I never had any—or menopause. That's one reason my weight has gone up, is because my condition has become worse as I hit perimenopause" (Wendy, 47, white). Wendy said that to manage the pain and to try to keep the illness from progressing, she swims every day. Swimming is a great form of exercise for someone who suffers from lipedema because it is low impact. Many people who have this condition are unable to exercise, and they are more likely to become immobile because of it.

One of the most devastating aspects of lipedema is the way people who suffer from it are treated. Sufferer's upper bodies are typically "normal" size, but their lower body is grossly distorted in size. Moreover, most physicians are not familiar with the disease and so they often recommend weight loss and blame it on poor eating habits and lack of activity. Unfortunately, if someone who is afflicted with lipedema does lose weight, they typically only lose it in their upper body, which makes their body look even more disproportional. People who suffer from lipedema endure the consequences of hyper(in)visibility because their ailment is hyperinvisible to most physicians and the public and their bodies frequently become hypervisible because they are often terribly disproportioned. In an attempt to help educate people about lipedema, Catherine Seo created a short documentary about the disorder in which she interviews physicians and sufferers from around the world.[7] Seo's documentary is an attempt to bring some much-needed visibility to an illness that is chronically invisible. In Western cultures, we have become so conditioned to the idea that fat is unhealthy that it is extraordinarily difficult to see a fat person without assuming that they are also unhealthy and that their body size is the result of poor lifestyle choices.

The Guise of Health

For many of the women I spoke with, they and their loved ones had a difficult time separating weight and appearance from health. As I discussed in Chapter 3, it was common for women to tell me that their mothers, grandmothers, or fathers often couched concerns about their weight in terms of their health, but most thought it was obvious that their family members were more concerned with their appearance: "They were always concerned about my health. The person that I probably got the most comments from was my grandma, but it was always—it was always under the guise of health. But every time I'd see her, she'd have some new diet article, or some new fitness thing, or whatever" (Pam, 29, white).

Family members put tremendous social pressure on most of these women to lose weight. They often made them feel that if they did not lose weight they would be unhealthy, or worse, die young because of their weight. But as I showed in Chapter 3, when some of the women resorted to extraordinarily unhealthy means to lose weight, they were applauded. In other words, it seems that the issue was with their appearance and not their health, or family members would have expressed concern about the manner with which they were losing weight. It was not just family members, though. Some of the women I interviewed also used the guise of health to discuss their appearance anxieties.

Liz gets straight to the point. She admits that her weight-loss desires have little to do with health. Of course, this could partially be because she is only 19. "I guess health is underlying, but for me, it's mainly because of looks. I'm very . . . I'm not very confident with how I look, obviously. I don't . . . the majority of my life I didn't like pictures; I refused to be in pictures. I was told—my mom told me if I wasn't in pictures, how would people know I existed? I was like, 'That's great'" (Liz, 19, white). A few minutes after this statement, she said she was working to become healthier and lose weight by going to the gym and eating better. She said, "I obviously get out of breath more easily than others." I asked her why this was "obvious" and she told me that it is because she is fat. Note that she also thinks it is "obvious" that she is not confident with how she looks. For Liz, it is readily apparent that a fat person is unhealthy (becomes easily winded) and is insecure or lacking in self-confidence. Fat marks the body as unhealthy and the person as having low self-confidence or self-esteem.

Patricia also attributes her being out of breath to her weight, but as she was talking with me about wanting to be healthier, she finished her thought with a reference to her appearance:

Healthy for me would be a reasonable weight. And I'm not, oh, I've got to get to 129.5 pounds. But certainly, for me, something that is in keeping with height/weight proportionate. I'm not talking supermodel. I'm not even talking wearing a bikini, just a good generally healthy weight and feeling better. I mean, I know. I'm winded. I walk across the parking lot, and I'm like, really? Seriously? You know? I know when my ankles can no longer support my weight. I watch my lower legs and calves swell up every day . . . but I'm motivated to lose the weight, but I'm also . . . I don't like what I see in the mirror. It's an ugly form. (Patricia, 47, white)

It was incredibly difficult for many of the interviewees to separate weight from health and appearance. The hypervisibility of the "obesity epidemic" coupled with the barrage of images of flawless women in popular culture perpetuates the idea that fatness signifies ill health and ugliness. These messages are so deeply entrenched in the cultural ethos that hardly anyone challenges or critiques them, including many of those who work in the health-care fields (Campos 2004; Cogan and Ernsberger 1999).

The Clinical Gaze

Physicians and health professionals in general constitute a fairly fatphobic group (Joanisse and Synnott 1999; Rand and MacGregor 1990). Numerous interviewees told me that their physicians reinforced the popular discourse that those who are fat are so because they are lazy and irresponsible (see also Campos 2004; Saguy and Riley 2005). Health-care workers are exposed to the same social messages about fat as the general population, so it is not surprising that they, too, would hold antifat attitudes. Yet the evidence suggests that negative attitudes expressed by medical professionals are directed not just toward "obesity" as a health condition but also against people who are fat (Schwartz et al. 2003; Teachman and Brownell 2001).

Part of the reason that many of the women I spoke with avoided going to the doctor was because they felt like no matter what their symptoms were, their size would be to blame. Interviewees lamented that when physicians only focused on their size and not the problem at hand, they felt like their real concerns were undermined and rendered hyperinvisible. Barbara told me a story about physician overlooking a blood clot:

> She missed so many things. I had a blood clot. It took an oncologist, when I was getting my mammogram, she told me you have cancer and you have some swelling in your leg, that's a sign of a blood clot. You need to go over right now. I had been telling my other doctor about it. Not good, they blame so much on your weight and I don't think they take in to account what you're saying to them at all. Just going to the doctor, there's so many things. You can't fit in the chair in the waiting room. You can't climb up on their table. They don't listen or they just jump to the weight instead of looking at the big picture. (Barbara, 45, white)

Barbara clearly demonstrates her frustration when she says that physicians do not listen or that they become hyperfocused on weight rather than the issues the patient is presenting.

Fernanda, whom I introduced previously, said, "It's a nightmare. They treat you like shit. [laughter] They treat you like shit. I used to cry every day." She laughed as she was telling me, but she also made it clear how traumatizing it was to be pregnant as a fat woman. She knew she felt good and was eating well, but every time she went to the doctor, they filled her with fears that she was going to develop gestational diabetes or have some other catastrophic health problem during the pregnancy.

Brooke was similarly negative about her experiences with physicians. She noted that she is healthy and it irritates her that doctors assume something is wrong with her or will be wrong with her soon because of her weight: "It makes me uncomfortable. I dread going to the doctor. I dread it. It's like, 'Oh shit, we're going to have to go through this again.' I'm a vegetarian. I go to the gym. My blood pressure's a little high, but that's genetic. Everything else is like completely perfect so why are you going to get on me about this? It's just ridiculous" (Brooke, 35, white).

The women I interviewed were not monolithic in their views about the relationship between weight and health. Yet almost all of them had had some sort of negative encounter with a physician or other health-care worker. Shawna said, "I had four babies in the hospital. I was treated pretty shitty by doctors and nurses along the way. My first was an old-school obstetrician. I had a pretty traumatic delivery with my first. He induced me early because he said the baby was big. I was pushing. He didn't even come over to me. He stayed at the doorway and was like, 'These aren't efficient pushes. We're going to need forceps'" (Shawna, 34, white). Shawna, pregnant with baby number six when we spoke, did not have her fifth baby in the hospital and was not going to have her sixth in the hospital either. She arranged home births and sought out midwives after having four negative experiences. She made it clear that the combination of the medicalization of childbirth with the medicalization or healthicization of fat was toxic for her and that she wanted her birthing experiences to be memorable and filled with joy.

Fernanda and Shawna were not the only two women who spoke about negative experiences during pregnancy; most of the women I interviewed who had children while fat experienced similar treatment. Those who did not have children were frequently reminded by their gynecologists that they needed to lose weight if they wanted to conceive and have a "normal" pregnancy.

In the clinical setting, fat women are hyper(in)visible to healthcare providers because fat has been medicalized rather than attributed to natural human variation. The providers see fat as a disease and discount the patient's symptoms or reduce any and all symptoms to their body weight. This situation is further exacerbated when patients who are fat are too large for the medical equipment, gowns, wheelchairs, and gurneys.

Too Big to Treat

In Chapter 2, I discussed situations where interviewees experienced anxiety and sometimes humiliation because they could not fit in restaurant booths, chairs, or other public spaces. Owen (2012) discussed the exclusion of fat people in society as a form of microaggression—a form of subtle discrimination. However, these subtle forms of discrimination can add up to disastrous consequences when it involves someone's health. Becky has sarcoidosis, but she will not go to the doctor because she is too large for the medical equipment and cannot take the emotional toll of being chastised and stigmatized for her weight:

> It's been an embarrassment. You know, and I don't even go to the doctor anymore. I don't go to the doctor anymore because, number

one, I can't fit into the chairs in the office. And like with my sarcoid disease, they need to take x-rays of my leg, my back, my chest—can't fit into the machines. They went to do an MRI. I was told, you know, to lay down on the table, then when they found that I was like 450 pounds, they said, "OK, you're going to have to get up off the table before it breaks. You're just too big. We can't get the scan on you." You know, so I sat there for a whole hour and a half for nothing. So it's just—it's an embarrassment, you know, and then people automatically assume you're just fat because you're just eating, eating, eating, eating, you know, too lazy to exercise, without even asking. (Becky, 32, African American)

Becky is embarrassed because she cannot fit on the standard MRI and x-ray equipment and is tired of having her time wasted because health-care providers cannot accommodate her body. She is also sensitive to the fact that the staff and clinicians assume that she is fat because she eats too much and does not exercise. The pervasive assumption that fat people overeat contributes to the stereotypes many hold about people who are fat. She is painfully aware of the hyper(in)visibility of her body in these contexts—her body is magnified while her needs are erased.

Kathryn told me a story about her experiences with a health-care provider who rendered her hyper(in)visible when their scale could not accommodate her weight:

> But their scale only went up to—I want to say 350 pounds, and I knew I weighed more than that, so they had to put me on a special scale in the bathroom, and I don't think they handled that very well, because the woman who was charged with taking my weight didn't know how to work the special scale, and she kind of—I was sort of standing in the hallway, and there was a conversation—I mean, it was back behind the doctor's door, so it wasn't in the waiting room, but you know, there was some conversation about how to use the scale, and kind of loud, so everybody could hear it, and I did put something on a comment card about that, because I didn't think it was appropriate. (Kathryn, 48, white)

Kathryn is both hypervisible and hyperinvisible in this situation, because weighing her became a spectacle as the nurse talked loudly about not knowing how to use the "special" scale. In addition, the staff was insensitive to the fact that having to be weighed on a "special" scaled could lead to embarrassment—her feelings were discarded.

Cathy also wondered aloud if those in the medical field even take into consideration the fact that some patients are excluded from testing and procedures because of their size: "There is always that kind of thought . . . do they consider people my size? I don't know. You never know if they've taken that into account. I mean I've had problems with when I had a MRI when I had those types of tests done, the tables were really small or I've been really smashed into little things that obviously weren't made for somebody my size" (Cathy, 44, white).

Cathy expresses the discomfort that she has experienced being "smashed" into a device that is too small to accommodate a large body. Cathy was able to have the procedures done, whereas Rita, who has anal cancer, was unable to get the tests she needed at her local hospital (in a major city). She had to travel approximately 60 miles to a facility that could accommodate her size. She is understandably angry about the fact that fat bodies are hyperinvisible when it comes to health care: "I've got news for you, if you're over 400 pounds and you get cancer you just better pay up your funeral bill, honey, because you're dead because it won't hold you. There's nothing they have to offer you. Unless you go home to starve yourself to get below 400 pounds, you can kiss their ass. You're not getting on it" (Rita, 59, white). Rita and others I talked with were frustrated with the fact that while there is unending attention paid to "obesity" and the emphasis on the increasing numbers of people who are "obese," there is still little offered when it comes to accommodations in health care—this is yet another predicament of the phenomenon of hyper(in)visibility.

As Rita indicated, sometimes the lack of accommodations or the stigma associated with fatness can lead to a person's death. For example, an emergency room physician by the name of Suzanne Dooley-Hash contributed a piece to the Binge Eating Disorder Association (BEDA) online newsletter about a patient whose death she attributed to weight stigma.[8] In the piece, Dr. Dooley-Hash describes a call she received from an emergency room physician "in the middle of nowhere" informing her that they were transferring a patient to her hospital—a five-hour trip by ambulance. When the patient arrived at her hospital, he was unconscious and barely breathing, but she later found out that when he arrived at the first hospital, he was talking and actually walked in on his own. The patient's sister begged Dr. Dooley-Hash to "not let him die just because he is fat." The sister told the doctor, "He's a good man." Initially Dooley-Hash did not understand the sister's pleas.

It turns out that the patient had a hole in his intestine and the reason he was transferred to her hospital was because the doctors at the first hospital did not want to operate on him because of his weight. The physicians at the first hospital argued that his quality of life was likely poor, the surgery was too risky because he was "morbidly obese," and he probably had other health problems. Of course, the surgeons had no evidence to indicate that his quality of life was poor or that he had other health problems. They assumed it because he was fat. Dr. Dooley-Hash's surgeons attempted surgery, but it was too late; he died. The patient's sister told Dooley-Hash how much he had dreaded going to the doctor because of the way he was treated by physicians. Dooley-Hash said she now understands why his sister insisted that her brother was a good man—despite his being fat. Technically, the cause of death was a perforated intestine, but according to Dr. Dooley-Hash, he died from weight stigma.

As I discussed previously, merely seeing a fat person is often evidence that there is something wrong with them, and frequently assumptions are made about the person's life. The surgeons at the first hospital thought that they knew something about this man simply based on his body weight, and their inaction, according to Dr. Dooley-Hash, cost a man his life. Not all fat persons are unhealthy or have a poor quality of life. In fact, many are quite fit.

Fit and Fat

"Fatness" and "fitness" are not typically two words that we hear in common association because of the assumption that if someone is fat, then he or she is not fit. Many of the women I spoke with were also surprised that they were healthy or fit even though they are fat. In the last decade, researchers have begun finding that not all fat persons are unhealthy. In the medical literature, this is referred to as the "obesity paradox" (Fleischmann et al. 1999). In fact, some fat persons are protected from various diseases and death because of their adipose tissue (Lainscak et al. 2012). Research has shown that some people in the "obese" category of BMI are protected from coronary artery disease (Cassuto et al. 2013), acute and chronic heart failure (Patsa et al. 2013; Pingitore et al. 2007), stroke and death following a stroke (Fonarow et al. 2007), certain types of cancers (Halabi, Small, and Vogelzang 2005), and chronic kidney disease (Fleischmann et al. 1999; Kalantar-Zadeh et al. 2005).

According to Campos et al. (2006), "obesity" and being "overweight" has been exaggerated as a risk factor and erroneously portrayed as causing poor health and morbidity (see also Burgard 2009, 49). Moreover, research clearly indicates that health risks, for people of all sizes, are lowered by physical activity, good nutrition, access to health care, and strong support networks, regardless of whether the person loses weight (Lamarche et al. 1992; Bjorntorp et al. 1970). However, interviewees and their physicians often framed their good health in terms of luck that could run out any day. They and their doctors were "amazed," "shocked," and "surprised" that they were in good health: "I remember, like, when I would go to a regular exam or something and they would be shocked my cholesterol was low, shocked that my blood pressure was fine. It was like you are bigger so we expect you to have high blood pressure and high cholesterol and it's really surprising, that kind of attitude" (Cathy, 44, white). Cathy's doctor was surprised that she had both low cholesterol and normal blood pressure, because she is "bigger" and health-care professionals assume that someone who is "obese" is also unhealthy. Krista demonstrated similar thinking when I asked her about her health:

JG: How is your health?
Krista: Surprisingly good.
JG: Yeah? And why do you say surprisingly?
Krista: Because you . . . and this is not you, but in general you would associate somebody that weighs 268 pounds with somebody that has a lot of health problems, but I don't have any health problems right now and hopefully it stays that way. (Krista, 28, white)

Krista is only 28 years old, but she still thinks it is surprising that she is currently in good health and is "hopeful" that she will stay that way. And Sue, who is 62 years old, said, "I am not diabetic. I am pretty lucky, considering, and at 62." Sue believes that a fat woman who is 62 years old is very lucky not to have diabetes or other major health problems. Yet healthiness was assumed to be a temporary state, because many of these women and their physicians thought that their weight would eventually begin to cause health problems.

Some of the women I spoke with were working tirelessly to lose weight by eating a low-calorie diet and exercising:

> I have a doctor that I see here regularly, every other appointment we do blood work on everything, and he was really shocked the first time I went in and did the blood work. He felt there has to be something. I'm eating a 1200-calorie diet. I'm active this much, and I'm not losing the weight. What am I not doing? He said, "Let's do a full blood work-up and we'll see." He came back and said, "There's no reason why you are not losing weight. You are healthy and everything. All of your levels are within normal. It's not slightly below normal. Everything was good, your cholesterol, everything. According to your blood work, you're not fat. In your blood work, it's not there." (Katrina, 31, white)

Katrina's physician seems to be unable to accept that a fat person can be healthy. His statement that "according to your blood you're not fat" is so telling regarding the predominant view among physicians. Katrina is fat and she is not experiencing any negative health consequences as a result of her body size, but both she and her physician are perplexed that she is not losing weight. Her blood work is probably good because she is incredibly active (Katrina is a fitness instructor and member of a belly-dancing troupe that performs regularly). Research shows that fitness is the key to optimal health (Ortega et al. 2012).

As is clearly indicated in these statements, some of the women I spoke with agreed with the dominant view that fat causes ill health, but there were other women I spoke with who seemed to understand that body weight does not determine one's health: "Because there are a lot of people who are never going to look like Christy Brinkley, who are very healthy. I mean, my doctor is still absolutely amazed every single time I see him. He's like, 'Your blood pressure is perfect.' I mean, I'm not the healthiest person on Earth, but I'm not dying either. I mean, I think people need to understand that not everyone is going to be 105 pounds" (Ann, 33, white). Ann points out that weight variation is normal and that people who are not "model thin" can also be healthy. She wants "people" (physicians, media, the general public) to understand that it is possible to be fit and fat.

Similarly, Sophia and Tracey both indicated that their body size does not dictate their health status:

> Truthfully, I'm pretty healthy. I mean, I've got some physical things going on, but I'm not diabetic and not prediabetic. All my lipids are good. My blood pressure is good. (Sophia, 55, white)

> I've never called in fat to work. I've never called in because my knees hurt. I never had any kind of issue related to my weight that kept me from doing my job or making me less productive. However, when I was a smoker, a pack a day smoker, I called in sick a lot because I would get bronchitis three times a year. Or I would develop a chest infection and not be able to come in and do my job. (Tracey, 32, white)

Sophia has a positive attitude and regards herself as "pretty healthy," especially compared to other people her age. And as Tracey indicated, weight does not prevent her from doing her job or other things that she finds enjoyable. She says that she has never "called in fat," but she did miss work when she was a smoker. Tracey's weight does not prevent her from being a "good citizen" in the neoliberal context, because despite her fat, she is able to participate in the labor force.

Health at Every Size®

Not all of the women I spoke with were "surprised" that they were in good health or thought that it was impossible to be healthy and fat. In fact, numerous women I spoke with subscribed to the Health at Every Size® (HAES) ideology.

Linda Bacon (2010) argues in *Health at Every Size* that the intent of HAES® is to help people shift their focus from hating their body and self to learning to accept and appreciate their body and life—regardless of their weight. She informs readers that HAES® is not speculation or unproven theory but rather is based on numerous scientific studies (p. 1). HAES® is based on size and self-acceptance, health enhancement, eating well, exercising for pleasure, and ending size discrimination (Burgard 2009). Bacon subscribes to "setpoint theory," the idea that each of us has a weight (plus or minus a few pounds) that our bodies will naturally gravitate to if we follow our internal cues of hunger and satiety. Many women I interviewed, especially from the first set of interviews, either had read Bacon's book or had encountered HAES® through online sources. Cathy explained, "So I'm trying to focus on that sort of just, I know being bigger doesn't make me feel better as far as fibromyalgia goes, so I'm just trying to focus on eating healthy, eating a whole foods diet and focusing on that. Eating when I'm hungry, stopping when I'm not hungry. Eating what I want to eat whenever I feel like my body is telling me to eat and seeing where . . . because I have no idea where my body weight is naturally right now. I've been all over the place" (Cathy, 44, white). Cathy's quote captures the premises of HAES®, and more specifically, she indicates that she also believes in setpoint theory. She is trying to listen to her body and eat when she is hungry so that her weight will eventually be "where it's supposed to be" according to her setpoint.

Nicole, who also has some mixed feelings about recent weight loss, is inspired by the HAES® model because it is not about trying to reach some lofty goal or trying to achieve a body size or shape that might never be possible. Instead, it is about taking care of her body and self and not emphasizing body size. Nicole told me, "In a way it [HAES] really inspires me to work out and feel good about myself. Like try to focus on . . . My roommate and I last night were talking about focusing on what your body can do rather than what your body looks like" (Nicole, 25, white).

HAES® is difficult to practice in a culture that bombards us with images of thin, beautiful women and fat-shaming messages and that tempts us with a cornucopia of heavily processed, high-fat, high-sodium, quick, cheap, and easy-to-prepare foods. According to the women I interviewed, listening to one's internal hunger cues and following bodily cravings is extraordinarily challenging, because they have spent most of their lives trying to suppress their hunger so that they could lose weight:

> Yeah, the tricky part is to have a good relationship with food. To eat when you're hungry, stop when you're full, and eat a variety of foods. Once you do that, and you know—exercise somewhat. Find something that's active that you enjoy. I'm not a big proponent of going to the gym and spending an hour on a treadmill and hating every minute of it—you feel like a hamster. Like I just try to move frequently. I just started a Yoga class. I'm really enjoying that. And I figure, you know, once I can normalize my relationship with food completely, whatever size I am is whatever size. I don't care if it's 200 pounds. I don't care if it's 240 pounds. I don't care if it's 140 pounds, although I'm really not thinking that's what it's going to be. My body will do what my body is supposed to do, and that's the end of that. (Carol, 30, white)

Carol wants to normalize her relationship with food, but she knows that this is the most difficult part because she has spent nearly her entire life regarding food as the enemy and cause of her problems. Now she is trying to shift her view and eat a varied but healthful diet. Rather than starving herself, she eats when she is hungry and is teaching herself to stop when she is full.

Susan is also focusing on her health and getting away from judging herself and her health by the number on the scale. Susan has other health conditions that require the regular use of the steroid prednisone, which causes fluid retention and weight gain. "Right now, I weigh about 260. I'm trying to just emphasize health, not weight, because I don't feel like I'm ever going to be a slim person. It's just not in my genetic makeup to be a slim person, plus the prednisone and everything else. I try to work out on my treadmill when I can, because I feel better, and that does help to keep the weight from ballooning too far out of control, and right now, I'm really kind of fortunate" (Susan, 46, white). Susan knows that she is not going to be "slim," but she also does not want to resign herself from feeling well. As Deb Burgard (2009, 44) said, "HAES defines health by the process of daily life rather than the outcome of weight." Unfortunately, this is not the hegemonic view of health—yet. There is increasing awareness of HAES® in the biomedical community, so perhaps the views will shift in time.

Conclusion

The neoliberal focus on health (especially the assumption that thinness signifies health) perpetuates the hyper(in)visibility of fat women. The women I interviewed demonstrated that what constitutes health in their eyes is complicated by the messages we as a society receive about the dangers of "obesity" and the "obesity epidemic." Most of the women expressed mixed views about whether or not they were healthy. They often said things like, "Overall I'm in good health, but I need to lose weight to improve my health." Statements such as these indicate that it is difficult to set aside the predominant messages about health from the larger culture, even when their own corporeal experiences tell them otherwise.

The stories these women shared about how they have been treated within the health-care system is consistent with what other researchers have found but are nonetheless disturbing (Tischner 2013). Research has shown that mistreatment, stigma, and discrimination lead to physiological problems (Muennig 2008). Marilyn Wann has discussed the "nocebo effect" of fat for years. A "nocebo" is a harmless substance that creates a powerfully harmful effect. In other words, being told that fat causes poor health or other conditions can actually make a fat person more likely to develop that condition. As Golda Poretsky says on her blog post about the nocebo effect, "The power of suggestion, is, well powerful."[9] Moreover, the harmful effects of the phenomenon of hyper(in)visibility are perpetuated when physicians attribute any and all health ailments to participants' size—their body is hypervisible—while simultaneously rendering participants' knowledge of their own bodies and symptoms hyperinvisible.

Hyper(in)visibility is further reinforced when equipment, gowns, and medical screening devices cannot physically accommodate the body of larger persons. This can lead to inadequate medical treatment or, worse, an untimely death. Medical schools should teach about the "obesity paradox" and the fact that "obesity" or weight in general is not simply the result of a single factor but rather a complex combination of lifestyle, genetics, environment, psychological health, and so forth. Perhaps the HAES® paradigm will become more readily accepted by persons in the biomedical community.

However, the recent move by AMA to label "obesity" a disease does not bode well for changing the hegemonic view of fat.

Now that fat has officially been designated a disease, there are concerns that other health conditions, like in Claudialee's case, will be overlooked and that increasing numbers of people will be misdiagnosed or have their actual diagnosis delayed. Others fear that the disease label will exacerbate what is quite frequently a tense relationship between people of size and their physicians—not to mention that the disease label could be used to prevent people of size from working in various industries or even adopting a child. Those who favor the disease label argue that it will provide protections to fat persons because the stigma associated with "obesity" will decrease because it will no longer be considered the fault of the individual person. Only time will tell how the official disease classification will affect actual persons. Regardless of the disease label, it was clear that the majority of the women I spoke with do not feel that they receive adequate treatment from health-care professionals.

Chapter 5

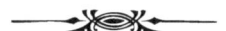

Ample Sex

The Illusion of a Paradox

Fat women are frequently considered deviant because they violate one of the most fundamental gender norms of Western culture: Women should be beautiful, or at least try, and fat is not typically considered beautiful. Depictions in the media of fat women as sexual are hardly common. In fact, the words "fat" and "sexy" are seldom used in the same sentence. Large women are often considered either nonsexual or sexually insatiable and desperate (Boero 2012; LeBesco 2004; Millman 1980; Prohaska and Gailey 2009). Of course, these are stereotypes. Nevertheless, there is a lack of scholarly literature[1] that focuses specifically on fat women's sexual experiences (for exceptions, see Gailey forthcoming, 2012; Murray 2004).

Fat represents a challenge to the identification as sexual (Murray 2004) because body size is connected to the heteronormative system of meaning and value that establishes what it means to be masculine and feminine. Heteronormativity is the assumption that humans are naturally heterosexual, and it prioritizes men's pleasure in sex. The Western configuration of the gender order, typically referred to as "hegemonic masculinity" (Connell 1987), is the blueprint for the way men should behave and the goals to which they should aspire, in addition to the type of women they should be attracted to, date, or marry. It is common, in this context, for men to dominate other men and subordinate women. Women are expected to accommodate the interests and needs of men, a concept known as "emphasized femininity" (Connell 1987), which includes meeting the normative standards of beauty (thinness). Emphasized femininity plays an important role in sustaining hegemonic masculinity and heteronormativity. "The fat female body is frequently not considered to align with the feminine ideal because it symbolizes domination or resistance to idealized femininity and overconsumption" (Gailey 2012, 116). Fat women's bodies tend to demonstrate characteristics associated with both masculinity and femininity. Their bodies are masculine because they take up a large amount of space, and their bodies are ultrafeminine because they are soft, curvy, and fleshy. By virtue of its size, the fat female body is simultaneously nonsexual and hypersexual (Braziel 2001; Lupton 2012).

To view fat women as both hypersexual and nonsexual suggests an interesting paradox. I argue that the phenomenon of hyper(in)visibility positions fat women at these two extremes. In other words, fat women are relegated by the culture and relegate themselves, through the embodiment of fat hatred, to the status of hyper(in)visible. Due to the tremendous amount of attention in the media and popular culture about the harms of fat, coupled with the constant barrage of highly sexualized images of thin, scantily clad women, we begin to associate sex and sex appeal with a specific body type. The illusion of a paradox reinforces the status quo. If we believe that someone cannot be both hypervisible and hyperinvisible, or nonsexual and excessively sexual, then it is easier to write off the observation and assume it is illogical or anomalous. But hyper(in)visibility is not anomalous; it is the norm and it buttresses the idea that fat women are deviant. So fat is a threat to masculinity and femininity because fat women who enjoy sex and find and pursue partners demonstrate that the conventional beauty messages are inaccurate or misleading.

The "fat is bad, thin is good" dichotomy is the dominant cultural frame for the discussion of health, beauty, and sexuality. The concept of framing refers to a strong tendency toward a preferred reading of events or issues reported (Goffman 1974). The media draw on culturally available frames when presenting stories to the public, which may influence people's judgments about attractiveness, health, or socially acceptable bodies. Media frames typically cast individuals as heroes or villains and center on issues of intention and motivation. The dominant frame emphasizes individual responsibility and generally avoids "structural level causes" (Saguy 2013). The prevailing discourse suggests that we have control over our bodies, that fat is unhealthy, and that individuals have a moral responsibility to lose weight. In other words, people are fat because they lack willpower or tenacity. Following this same line of thinking, women of size are responsible for their failure to meet societal norms and they are at fault if they are mistreated or stigmatized. Locating blame on fat women presumes that staying fat is a choice.

This dominant frame is not only apparent in the media; it is also quite popular among scholars.[2] Susie Orbach argues in her book *Fat Is a Feminist Issue* that women overeat and gain weight to hide their bodies from the male gaze. In essence, fat women intentionally desexualize their bodies so that they are not sexually objectified. Orbach's assumption is that fat is not sexy and that fat women are not sexual. Moreover, women are assumed to have less control over their bodies and desires because their reproductive capabilities make them "closer to nature."

Feminists have argued that the connection between women and nature provides a justification for the oppression of women and the control and surveillance of women's bodies (Bordo 1993). As Boero (2012, 55) states, "This long-standing ideological framing of women's unpredictable nature plays itself out in their presumed disordered eating." Boero contends that women are blamed for the obesity epidemic because they are "unruly" and "out-of-control," and she argues that "at its most basic level, the obesity epidemic is about women" (Boero 2012, 55). The women featured in this book made numerous references to their "unruly appetites" and "out-of-control" bodies, and some of them spoke about their insatiable sexual desires, but for the most part, their narratives seemed to follow that of many women's sex lives, except that they had the additional burden of hyper(in)visibility.

In sum, the "obesity epidemic" has been framed as an issue that is "threatening our very existence,"[3] and fat women are frequently the target of hostility and blame. Their bodies are often deemed unsightly, unkempt ticking time bombs. This framing is hardly sexy. But they are also assumed to be incapable of managing their desires and, in turn, sexually desperate (Prohaska and Gailey 2009). I contend that this marginalized status contributes to and perpetuates mistreatment by sexual partners. Moreover, the embodiment or internalization of fat hatred contributes to the performance of hyper(in)visibility, where women of size position themselves as Other by engaging in stereotypical behaviors. In the remainder of the chapter, women's voices guide us through their dating and sexual histories and demonstrate how the phenomenon of hyper(in)visibility plays out in this aspect of their lives. In addition, I highlight the various techniques these women used to transgress the way they see their body and subvert some of the negative messages.

Hidden Desires

Research about men who have sex with fat women has tended to focus on fat admirers (those who prefer large women) and those who humiliate fat women in an attempt to achieve masculinity, a practice commonly referred to as "hogging." Fat admirers are sometimes "in the closet," meaning that they are reticent about their attraction to fat women probably because of the "courtesy stigma" (Goffman 1963) they are likely to receive as a result of their association with and attraction to fat women. Fat women are stigmatized, and as a result, those who are attracted to or who associate with a stigmatized person or group are often the recipients of a "courtesy stigma." Goode and Preissler (1984) and Swami and Tovée (2009) studied fat admirers and found that fat admirers tend to reject the cultural norms associated with beauty. However, the largest proportion of the men interviewed by Goode and Preissler were "closet" and not "overt" fat admirers (p. 180). Moreover, very few men identified as exclusively dating fat women, and those who are genuinely attracted to women of size may keep it a secret to avoid reprisal.

Hogging is a practice where men target women they deem fat for "sport" or sexual pleasure (Gailey and Prohaska 2006). When hogging happens in a group of men, it frequently involves a bet about who can "pick up" the largest woman. The goal is sex, but sometimes a dance or phone number from a fat woman will suffice. When Gailey and Prohaska (2006) asked one of their interviewees to describe how the men determined if their friend actually succeeded and won the bet, he explained that they sometimes engage in behaviors in which they humiliate the women they deem fat (cf. Flood 2008). For example, both Gailey and Prohaska's and Flood's participants discussed a "rodeo." A rodeo takes place when a man's friends hide in the room where the couple is having sexual intercourse. When the friends think the couple is "really into it," they jump out of hiding and typically yell, snap pictures, and set a stopwatch to time how long their friend can hold on to the woman before she "escapes."

Other times, men reported that they engaged in hogging when they were "hard up" or horny and no one else was available to satisfy their sexual needs. After having sex with the woman, they tend to engage in bonding activities with their friends, such as bragging about how "she did whatever they wanted" and how easy or desperate she was, and sometimes they tell stories about how they mistreated her (i.e., calling her disparaging names or kicking her out of the car when they were finished). Gailey and Prohaska's (2006) participants indicated that they thought fat women were easy and desperate for attention because they assumed that the women were insecure (Prohaska and Gailey 2010, 2009). Of course, the men interviewed by Gailey and Prohaska denied hogging themselves because they had "standards," and they frequently stated that their friends who hog are sexually desperate, too.

Men who hog tend to avoid Goffman's "courtesy stigma" because they engage in hegemonic masculinity, where they denigrate the woman to her face or behind her back. In other words, under the script of hegemonic masculinity, sex is a conquest and a way to improve one's standing among other men. Men who hog are able to boost their social status because having sex with a fat woman is better than no sex, especially when they can joke about how easy she was or how despite mistreating her she still had sex with them—implying that they are sexually irresistible or some sort of "stud" (Gailey and Prohaska 2006; Prohaska and Gailey 2010). Most of the women I talked to knew about hogging, even though I did not ask them, and feared that men sometimes pursue large women because they think that such women are desperate.

Some of the women I interviewed expressed concerns that men targeted them on dating sites because they are fat and presumably lonely. For example, Meredith, 52 and white, talked about a man trying to swindle money out of her online. She described how convincing he was when he lied about his predicament and how he tricked both her and her adult daughter. When he asked for money, she said she knew he was trying to take advantage of her. But she said that in her younger days she might have fallen for it.

Two other women talked about feeling like men had sex with them because there was no one else around, because they were intoxicated, or because the men assumed that they were easy:

> They were drunk. I was definitely treated like the last pick, kind of. I never felt like they wanted to be with me. It was more like, "Well all the other girls are taken." I don't know if I felt that and projected it onto them, but it really seemed like that. (Elizabeth, 30, white)

> Well, I don't know. I got drunk—I was underage, and I got drunk, and I slept with a couple of guys that I never would have slept with had I been sober. And I think they only slept with me because they thought I was easy because I was heavy. You know, they would have never looked twice at me otherwise. (Janet, 36, white)

I asked Janet how she knew that they would not have paid attention to her, and she told me that she saw them both afterward and that the guys not only ignored her but tried to hit on her thin friends. Elizabeth recognized that she may have misperceived the men's intentions, but she was clear that they did not seem like they wanted to be with her while they were having sex. These statements also provide some perspective on the visibility of both of these women. Janet and Elizabeth became visible to the men when there was no one else around and the guys were drunk. If the men had not been drunk or if other (thinner) women had been around, both Elizabeth and Janet revealed that they probably would have remained invisible to these men.

The women I spoke with were aware that men play jokes on large women and were sometimes overly cautious because of this. However, it was also fairly clear that the women were sometimes interested in having sex and were looking for someone to validate them as sexually desirable. Even if they knew that some men would not be seen publicly with them, they also knew that they could fairly easily find a willing partner, even if just for one night.

Marked Shame

Social control of fat women's sexuality occurs through stigma, shaming, abuse, and victimization. Fat hatred is prolific in the United States. It seems as though the more attention that is paid to the "obesity epidemic," the more people fear fat or despise those who are fat. This is certainly related to the framing and discourse within which discussions about "obesity" take place. One of the concerns expressed about the "obesity epidemic" is that it costs the United States billions of dollars in health-care costs and lost wages. Some scholars have argued that fatphobia stems from an assumption that fat persons consume more than their share of the available resources (Farrell 2011). This is in addition to the dominant cultural frame that suggests that fat persons are capable of losing weight through hard work and that anyone who remains fat has chosen to be fat because they are lazy or undisciplined. These messages are proliferated throughout the culture, so it is not surprising that the majority of the women I interviewed also reported feeling disgusted by their own bodies and the bodies of other fat people.

When fat women do not feel desirable or attractive, they sometimes engage in regrettable behaviors or remain with partners who are abusive, because the women believe that they are undeserving of respect or proper treatment (cf. Royce 2009). Numerous women I interviewed discussed how they thought they had to endure mistreatment, lies, or disrespect because they assumed no one else would love them. For many of those women, this belief stemmed from remarks and comments that their parents, grandparents, or other highly influential adults in their life made when they were young, not to mention the insidious messages propagated through various forms of media about "unattractive" or "nonsexual" fat women.

Women in this study who internalized the message that fat is ugly or unattractive felt that their fat marked them as worthless or as less deserving of respectable treatment. In some instances, men used societal fatphobia against their partners through insults, verbal attacks on their desirability, and threats of leaving them or not going out into public with them (cf. Royce 2009).

Cassie's story about the first person she had sex with demonstrates both her and her partner's shame about her body:

Oh my God, this is the first person who's ever seen me naked, the first person that I've done anything sexual with and the idea that . . . the other part that made the relationship completely fucked up, the biggest part to me that I'm probably still dealing with the repercussions ten years later is that he was completely ashamed of me. He liked bigger girls, but I was the biggest he'd been with and he didn't even want to be seen in public with me. I didn't meet any of his friends, I didn't meet his parents, I wasn't invited to his birthday parties, I wasn't invited to his graduation. It's funny I remember we started talking in a January and maybe three weeks later he told me, "I care about you already and I want to be with you, but I want to be with somebody who my friends find fuckable," essentially. (Cassie, 33, white)

He wanted to be with someone in public whom his friends would find attractive because that would boost his social status, whereas being seen with a fat woman would lower his social credibility, or even worse, he might receive a courtesy stigma for being with her. Cassie "put up with it" because she thought that she deserved this sort of treatment. She told me that she was ashamed of her body and believed that other people found her unattractive because of her body size. She thought that if she wanted to have a relationship with a man, she would have to make some compromises, and that included being with someone who was embarrassed to be seen with her.

Cassie was not the only woman who reported that men were hesitant to be seen in public with her. Nicole said, "It's hard to quiet that voice in your head that says, 'If you lost weight maybe someone would find you attractive,' attractive enough to be a public girlfriend or whatever." Nicole wants to date someone whom she can date in public, who wants to be seen with her, but she fears that as long as she is fat, she will not meet someone who will be seen with her: "I don't actually have that many problems being naked in front of someone that I know wants to have sex with me. It's interesting, I think there are a lot of people who would have sex with me, but I think that a lot of people may not want to date me because then you would have to tell all your friends that you're dating me" (Nicole, 25, white). Nicole, unlike some of the women I give voice to next, does not have a problem with her sexual partners seeing her naked. Her concern is finding someone who will be seen in public with her. Fears about living alone, never marrying, or finding someone who is attracted to them came from stories about hogging, family members who told them they would never be loved, and the larger cultural messages about what attractive women look like. As Koppelman states, "In a society with a general penchant for punishing difference, and an excessively high regard for bodily appearances as cultural markers, it makes perfect sense that fat bodies will be abused in a variety of ways" (Koppelman 2003, 258). The abuse that comes from physicians, strangers, family members, and loved ones perpetuates the idea, for many large women, that they are undeserving of love and respect and are unattractive.

Tina, a woman who is somewhat involved in size acceptance through her attendance at the yearly National Association to Advance Fat Acceptance (NAAFA) convention and through some performance art, discussed how she struggled in mainstream society because she was not seen as sexual. Men typically did not look at her as sexual and she felt like she was missing something that she really needed—to be seen as sexual. When she started attending NAAFA conventions and the dances they host, she finally found the attention she had been craving: "It was really important for me to have the attraction element, and it's different—you know, I weigh 500 pounds, and most men don't look at me as a sexual being. And at the convention [NAAFA], I am looked at that way. There is also the carrying it to the other extreme where you know, suddenly I'm an object, but you know, you just can't take everything personally" (Tina, 34, white). The attention at the NAAFA convention was at the other extreme. She was a sex object, but she found this preferable to being hyperinvisible and feeling like she should be ashamed of her appearance and body. And she was not the only woman I spoke with who reported getting a "high" from all the attention at convention dances and meet-ups. However, some women I spoke with specifically avoided the convention parties because of the objectification. They spoke about men coming to the dances exclusively to look at fat women, and some feared that they were fat fetishists or were only interested in having sex with large women. One participant who attended NAAFA dances with relative frequency when she was in her early twenties thought that most of the men in attendance were married and definitely "in the closet" about their attraction to fat women.

Respondents who attended NAAFA conventions were not the only ones to report being treated as objects. Margo told me the story about the first time she had sex. She reported feeling used and objectified, and she set aside her own needs and feelings in order to feel sexually attractive and desired:

> He and I had gone through a lot of stuff, like he knew a lot about all my insecurities and things like that, and he knew that I'd never really had sex before or anything, and so we had talked about it a lot, and I was like I don't want to meet you in person because I'm afraid you're not going to like me once you see what I really look like. So he had me send him pictures of myself, and eventually, I sent him nude pictures of myself, and he still at that point was like it's OK, it's all cool, you know, still want to get together, and then when he stopped talking to me, I assumed it was because he had decided he didn't like my pictures, because of course, that was the only thing that I could get—it didn't occur to me that there could be things going on in his life. So we finally got together, and I thought we were going to like go out or whatever, and I met him downstairs at the motel I was staying at, because I didn't want to meet him for the first time in my room. I didn't even know the guy. And so we met, and he hugged me and kissed me, and that was pretty cool. I was all excited about that, and then we went back up to my room, and he sat down, and he was like OK, what do we do now? And I was like I don't know what we do now, because I'm scared. I told you that. And basically, he was just like well, we're not going to do anything until you feel you want to. And so I had no idea. I was just totally embarrassed and humiliated and I had no idea what to say. So he sat there for about half an hour, and neither of us talked at all, and that was kind of excruciating. And then eventually, he was like OK, well, let's kiss, and so we did, and things progressed, and we ended up having sex. And he just, like, went to sleep, and then got up and left in the morning, and I didn't hear from him for like two months after that. (Margo, 30, white)

Margo's story demonstrates how body shame and fat hatred can affect women who are fat and their interactions with sexual partners. Margo had never had sex and she was reportedly not ready, but she was also extremely self-conscious and at every turn kept expecting that this man she met online was going to decide that she was too fat or too ugly to meet in person. She acquiesced at each stage of the interaction by doing things she had previously said made her uncomfortable. He made her think that he respected her wishes by saying that they were not going to do anything until she was ready, but then he sat next to her in silence. The silence, according to Margo, made her feel like the decision was not up to her; the decision had already been made. He was going to have sex with her and he wore her down by making her so uncomfortable and self-conscious that she eventually gave in when he suggested that they kiss after a half hour of silence.

Several women literally said to me during the course of the interview that even though they had never said it aloud before, in the back of their minds they thought they should not ask for too much from their partners because they were probably "lucky to get anything at all"—in essence, to have someone pay attention to them sexually. Their needs and desires remained hidden or invisible because they felt ashamed of their bodies. They believed what they had been told and acted accordingly. They did not see themselves as sexy or worthy of attention from those who would treat them well and who were genuinely interested in them.

Fortunately, not all the women I spoke with felt that way, but there was a sense that many of these women felt like they had to put up with mistreatment from their partners or settle for less than satisfactory sexual encounters because of their size (cf. Royce 2009). Bonnie discussed how she repeatedly dated men who had drug or alcohol problems and took advantage of her:

> I'd get up and go to work, and there'd be people up and in the house, and I'd come home from work, and there'd be people out in the house and the yard, and I'd go to bed, and there'd be people up and in the house and in the yard—and I just let Randy do whatever he wanted to. And, you know, I just didn't have any boundaries. I didn't have any strong sense of self when it came to men. In other areas of my life, I absolutely did, but when it came to men, I just—I just didn't. (Bonnie, 51, white)

Randy did not own the house, Bonnie did; not only that, but Randy was not paying rent or any of the household bills. Bonnie did not have a "strong sense of self" when it came to men because she felt like she was lucky to have a man around who *seemed* to be attracted to her or who wanted to be with her. Bonnie allowed Randy to take advantage of her. She erased her boundaries, not just with him, but with other men she dated, too.

In addition to having trouble establishing boundaries, undressing was difficult for some of the women who were ashamed of their body. As Claire, a 35-year-old white woman, noted, "The heavier I became, the more self-conscious, and I just felt like I wasn't—nobody would want to go out with me, and I was embarrassed to get naked or have sex." A few of the women also discussed difficulties undressing in front of their current partner because they thought that their partner would view their body the way they do—as unattractive. When I asked them what they were afraid of, they said that they thought their partner would be surprised to see their curvy flesh, feel their rolls, and see the dimples in their skin even if this was their long-term partner or someone with whom they previously had sex.

Elizabeth discussed concerns with where her partners touched her during sex. She also noted that she was so preoccupied with her body that she was unable to orgasm until she met her husband:

> *Elizabeth:* Where major rolls are or jiggling you don't squeeze the fat. You don't go . . . Like the belly is like an area of, "Oh, should I be self-conscious, like what is he doing?" Even my butt, it's so big, there's this big swooping action and I'm like, "Oh gosh, can we not do that." Or the sides where there's rolls and stuff like that. Those are areas that are just generally not touched so if they're going to be touched or if they're being touched then my mind spikes, "What is he thinking? Why is he touching me there? What is he thinking when he's touching me there? Does that gross him out?"
> *JG:* Is it hard to be sexually satisfied if you're concentrating on . . .
> *Elizabeth:* Oh yeah. I never, never, ever, ever, ever, came with any other guy. (Elizabeth, 30, white)

She described herself as "extremely sexual," and she has had numerous partners, so it is telling that she was not able to reach orgasm with anyone prior to her husband. She attributed it to the fact that she was self-conscious about her body—how her body felt to her lovers and what it looked like. Body image concerns play an important role in sexual pleasure and functioning for women (Wiederman and Hurst 2008). In fact, women who are more self-conscious also are more likely to be ambivalent in sexual decision making and risk taking (Sanchez and Kiefer 2007). Unfortunately, it is not surprising that women sometimes have sex with men who they think are using them or taking advantage of them if they are ashamed of their bodies and appearance.

REFLECTED ACTS

In addition to the assumption that fat women are not sexual or not attractive, the dating world is an arena where masculinity and femininity are played out and traditional gender roles are reinforced. Fearing rejection, many single women of size perpetuate traditional gender norms about men and women's roles in dating and sexual behaviors. They are not just "doing gender" (West and Zimmerman 1987); they are also "doing fat," which involves engaging in extreme femininity and the reinforcement and perpetuation of stereotypes about fat women. Recall from previous chapters that doing fat is an accomplishment, similar to doing gender, that emerges in social interactions and occurs when fat individuals, or formerly fat individuals who still see themselves as fat,[4] engage in behaviors that perpetuate or signify fatness. Just as those who do gender organize their activities to reflect or express gender and are disposed to see others' behaviors in a comparable fashion, doing fat also means that fat persons organize their actions to reflect or express being fat and see other fat persons similarly (West and Zimmerman 1987: 127). When the negative connotations associated with fat are internalized, women sometimes act according to those preconceived notions.

In the following accounts, both Shannon and Bonnie are doing fat as they discuss their concerns about the type of men who they think are likely to be attracted to them. Both desire a relationship and want men to find them attractive, but they are also concerned that something might be wrong with men who are attracted to fat women:

> And I do feel, like a bit, with my weight that maybe I have to lower my expectations, because I have to find someone who is willing to date me at my size, and so maybe there's something wrong with

them because they want to date me at my size, so I have to be able to be OK with that, you know? (Shannon, 33, African American)

On the one hand, there's a part of me that thinks I should be glad that someone would look at me and go, "Wow, she looks really attractive." But the kind of Catch-22 that I do in my own mind is well, "What's wrong with them if they do?" You know, because someone my size is outside of the norm, and is certainly outside of what you're bombarded with from the media every day and every minute, and so I kind of sometimes put myself between a rock and a hard place as far as being able to accept that someone would look at me and find me physically attractive, and want that, and yet not want that at the same time. (Bonnie, 51, white)

Shannon, an African American woman, talked about how difficult it is to find a partner who is equally educated, from a middle-class background, and who finds her attractive. She mentioned at another point in our conversation that she often feels like an outsider in the Black community because of the intersection of her high educational achievement, her size, and her social class background. She fears that she might have to lower her expectations because of her size, and she is worried that only men who have obvious flaws are attracted to large woman. Both Bonnie and Shannon are doing fat by expressing serious reservations about the type of men who are attracted to fat women and through their assumption that they might have to lower their expectations or "settle."

In the following account, Jennifer recalls her online dating experiences. She mentioned that she did not have much success until she met her current boyfriend and that she found the whole process rather unsettling. Jennifer said she rarely contacted men, partly because she was concerned about rejection but also because in her experience when she did contact them first, they typically did not respond. She attributed it to her size, because she said she was open and honest about her size in her profile. "And the rare occasions that I did try to message them, that was their out, like they wouldn't respond. So, it's like, my expectations are lowered just to my experiences. Like it was, it didn't just come out of nowhere like, that's what happened. So, my experience, my expectations adjusted accordingly" (Jennifer, 34, white). Jennifer thought she would have to lower her standards because the pool of men available who are attracted to fat women is limited, and she feared there would be even fewer available and interested men if she expected them to have a similar education level. Much to her surprise, she did not have to lower her standards. She described her boyfriend very lovingly and said that they are a good fit. She also expected that the six-month relationship would likely turn into marriage. Other women I interviewed who met smart, caring, loving men said that they hoped that all women of size would realize that they do not have to settle or put up with mistreatment.

According to my interviewees, men still largely control dating. While women are increasingly taking the initiative and pursuing men, according to the women I spoke with, it is still men who are "in control." For the most part, participants waited for men to contact them on Internet dating sites. It seemed that for some of the women this was exaggerated because they do not feel attractive. They expressed concern that men would use them, reject them, take advantage of them, avoid being seen in public with them, or objectify them. Fat women's bodies are deviant, according to the dominant cultural framework, so their actions cannot be; conformity to gendered expectations becomes even more important for women who are fat, because fat is a threat to both masculinity and femininity.

Three of the women were in exclusively same-sex relationships, and their concerns about the way their bodies looked were similar to those who identified as strictly heterosexual. For example, Brenda, who has been in a relationship with her partner for 25 years, said, "Well, I mean I see myself naked and it grosses me out. I mean I'm old and my spouse is older so that's not the issue, but then we don't have a very physical relationship and sometimes I wonder how much of it is because of the way I look. She says it's not, but well I think if I was prettier or thinner . . ." (Brenda, 51, Native American). Brenda thinks her body is gross because of her body size, and she assumes that her partner feels the same way. I asked if her partner was also a large woman and she said yes, but she still thought that their lack of physical intimacy was because of her body. Again, I only spoke with three women who are exclusively in same-sex relationships, but all three said they wanted to be pretty and sexy for their partners and all expressed concerns that their weight might be a turn off. Dawn, 34 and white, said that she thought appearance norms were changing in the lesbian community and that she has noticed more pressure on lesbians to meet conventional beauty norms, such as being thin, wearing makeup, and having stylish, more feminine hair.

Nine of the women in the sample identified as bisexual, and their experiences were not markedly different than the other women. Several spoke specifically about trying to meet partners and stated that they usually let both men and women approach them because they assumed that others would not find them attractive and they did not want to risk the embarrassment of rejection. According to these data, doing fat does not seem to be specific to heterosexual women. Doing fat, like doing gender, happens because of the expectations the culture and individuals have about "appropriate" behaviors for fat people; therefore there is no reason to expect that only heterosexual fat women do fat. However, numerous women found ways to subvert the dominant frame and challenge both gender and body norms.

Shifting Reflections

In a study published in the inaugural issue of *Fat Studies*, I found that women who came to embrace their fat bodies reported higher levels of sexual enjoyment than they did prior to accepting their body (Gailey 2012). Size acceptance is one avenue, but there are other ways that women find to accept their bodies and enjoy sex (see also Gailey forthcoming). Some of the paths that led to greater body acceptance involved experimentation and participation in alternative sexual lifestyles; involvement in activities such as belly dancing, massage therapy, and weight lifting; finding partners who love their bodies and made that known; or getting older. Embodiment of fat, or accepting and embracing one's fat body, involves a process whereby these women have found ways to make their bodies visible on their own terms:

> The impression I get is that people just think that large women, we're just lonely, and we're just by ourselves and don't really have anybody who is interested in us, and really I've found that there are so many people who are interested in women of larger proportions

because that's truly what they're attracted to, and just, you know, it's kind of sad to me when I see women who are the same way now that I was a couple of years ago, and just feeling bad about themselves and settling. It just sucks, because there's really no reason to settle. You have to go for what you want, find it, and that's kind of where I'm at now. I'm just so happy with my life, and it took me a long time to get there, but just so happy now. I have the best husband, and it's an alternative lifestyle, and it may not be for everybody, but it works for me, and I didn't settle for less than what I wanted. And I got it. (Veronica, 28, white)

Veronica's quote illustrates what many of the women communicated to me: there is no reason to settle for less, there is no reason to believe that there are not good people attracted to large women, and it is possible to have a happy, fulfilling relationship.

Of the 74 women, 16 engaged in alternative sexual lifestyles. Alternative sexual lifestyles included participation in BDSM (bondage, discipline, sadomasochism), polyamory (more than one lover), open relationships, and group or public sex. Seven women were actively involved in BDSM, 10 experimented with various forms of BDSM, 8 women identified as currently or previously involved in polyamorous relationships, and 9 women had engaged in public or group sex. There is some overlap in these categories: 3 women had engaged in all these sexual lifestyles, and 3 engaged in two of them. Just as being involved in the size acceptance community had a positive impact on some respondents' body image and sexual expressiveness, involvement in an alternative lifestyle relationship or finding the kink community had similar affects, according to the women I spoke with (Gailey forthcoming):

> I'm the one—you know, I mean, he listens to me, we're very—one of the things that you have to be in a D&S relationship is very—communication is very top notch. You have to talk about everything. You have to talk about, even after you play a scene, or do a scene, where he's in total control, and one of you is not in control. You know, you have to be able to talk about what did you like, what you didn't like, was it good, was it bad. You know? And, even on his side. He may not like what he did or didn't get the reaction he expected to get. So it's a very interesting dynamic to the relationship. And one of the books I highly recommend to people is *The*

Loving Dominant, for both submissive and dominants to read. But it's been an experience. It's been probably the most sexually satisfying relationship I've ever been in in my life. (Sally, 46, white)

Sally has found that involvement in a dominant and submissive relationship has helped her come to terms with her body and truly enjoy sex. Several interviewees mentioned that men and women of size are common in the kink community (cf. Newmahr 2011). Moreover, I was told that larger bodies are sometimes preferred in the kink community because of the presence that a large body demands:

> Being involved in the kink community since I've moved here has been so amazing for my body acceptance. It's huge, it's been huge, huge, and huge because back home my kink was all related to sex and I wasn't involved in community or anything like that. And then I moved out here and my roommate was involved in the kink community and she introduced me to people and took me to parties. And my first kink party I went to I'd never met these people before and my roommate said this guy was cool and that she was comfortable with me playing with him and he wanted to play with me and I was just like, OK. And it was funny, it was my first party, first time meeting these people, and I got completely naked in front of them and I was just like, oh my God. (Cassie, 33, white)

Cassie said that she was able to disrobe in this new group because she felt welcomed and that there were other people of size there. In Staci Newmahr's (2011) ethnographic book *Playing on the Edge: Sadomasochism, Risk, and Intimacy*, she discussed the role of weight in the kink community she studied. She described a community where a number of the members, both men and women, were "obese," but she stated that weight was not a salient part of the discourse. It was not that fatness was desired but that it was not stigmatized—it ceased to be a social marker. In this particular community, and others as described by my participants, fatness is not hyper(in)visible, which is partly why women in my study who participated in SM communities were able to better accept their bodies—this was one place where they were not Othered or marginalized.

There are additional ways that some of the women found to shift the way they see their bodies, such as through activities like massage therapy, belly dancing, and exercise. "I'm at a place of peace for once. As part of becoming a massage therapist, I got the opportunity to work through a lot of the I-hate-my-body stuff, and actually connect in with my body, which was a glorious experience—incredibly challenging, but glorious. I feel pretty good" (Tina, 34, white). Tina had a history of disassociating from her body. She even talked about not realizing she had a sprained ankle because she was so "out of touch" with her body. When Tina started massage therapy classes, she had to allow people to touch her, and she learned how to connect with her own body. She has quit denigrating herself and stopped focusing on what she would like to change about her appearance. Instead, she now focuses on what feels good and what she needs. Her body is visible in her mind and she accepts it as part of her, not a separate entity or object of revulsion.

Katrina also described finding an activity that has helped her not only improve her fitness level but also change the way she sees her body. She started belly dancing and was eventually invited to join a belly-dancing troupe. After a while, she and a friend began their own belly-dancing troupe and started performing all over, including at the state fair: "We are good enough, and we keep the crowd entertained, I think. We aren't bad-looking girls. It's just one of those things where it has really improved the way I think of myself. It doesn't change the fact that I would like to be smaller, but I don't have a desire to be a tiny girl. My ideal body is a size 16, 18 somewhere in there" (Katrina, 31, white). Katrina would like to lose weight, but performing as a belly dancer has helped her self-esteem tremendously, because people complement her on how good she is and how beautiful she is. Belly dancing has provided a space for her to be visible without being Othered. Katrina is a large woman, and she said she knows that she will never be small. However, she is much more realistic about her goals, and she now appreciates what her body does for her and she does not feel as unattractive as she did prior to learning to belly dance.

Exercise was tremendously helpful for many women when it came to getting in touch with their bodies and feeling better, as Kathryn's statement indicates:

> I feel pretty good. I get frustrated because I think there is so much conflict between how I feel about myself, and how the larger society

does. I'm probably midsize fat, you know, like a size 22–24, but especially like the last six months, I've been lifting weights, like I'm really strong underneath all my fat. I feel like I'm a really well built sofa. I've got a really strong frame with all this nice cushioning padding, and I just don't understand why larger society doesn't see that as a positive, you know, as a positive variation in how bodies are built. I'm healthy. I'm functional. You know, I'm kind of cute, but I don't think that that's—I don't think that's typical for someone to feel good in a body like mine. (Kathryn, 48, white)

She is healthy, cute, and disappointed that our society sees her as an ugly, unhealthy woman with low self-esteem. The projected image about the way that women who are fat are supposed to behave and feel is often in conflict with the way the women actually do feel and behave. Unfortunately, it takes a lot of work and willpower to overcome the dominant cultural frame and feel good about a body that is marginalized and despised.

Loving, adoring partners provide a fabulous path toward feeling better about one's body. For some women, it was their husband or partner who helped them find beauty in their bodies, but for others it was a less serious sexual relationship. For Tracey, a woman who was in a reportedly lifeless marriage, the body image boost came from someone she was friends with and had not seen in a number of years:

> I wanted to know if he was attracted to me. As it turns out he was, and eventually we started to flirt with each other in not-so-subtle ways, and he made me feel like the most incredibly sexual and beautiful woman he ever laid his eyes on. I'd never felt that way before. I didn't know that it was possible to feel completely idolized by another person. I had no idea. I had no idea that it was possible to be a sex object for somebody and to have him fantasize about me and to dream about me and to masturbate at the thought of me. What? Really? Is this my life? (Tracey, 32, white)

The man she described became her lover and they are now cohabitating, but the account is how she remembers the beginning of their affair. She finally felt like she was visible to someone she was attracted to, and it made her feel alive and wanted, unlike how she felt for years when she assumed that no one would find her attractive, let alone fantasize about her.

Another woman whom I interviewed is a cancer survivor, and she explained how she and her partner (now husband) learned to cope with the fact that her treatment for anal cancer left her unable to have vaginal intercourse. He not only cared for her while she was going through intense chemotherapy and radiation but has remained by her side, and they were married a few months before we spoke:

> He's had to live with the fact that we can't be sexual in a traditional sexual way anymore. He's had to take care of me a lot and he gladly does it. He just loves my fat belly. He goes to sleep in my fat arms and finds it very comforting. He doesn't know why he likes that; he's known since he was in elementary school that he was always interested in the fat girls. I think for him, while he would certainly like a thick woman, what a black man calls a thick woman, he prefers a supersized woman. He likes the belly. He likes big arms and not in a sexual way. I think it's very comforting to him. He likes it sexually; don't get me wrong, but . . . (Rita, 59, white)

Rita's new husband is also 16 years younger than her, but he has shown her that he loves her, and they have found new ways to be intimate. In fact, when he proposed, he told her that he did not think there was anyone he could be more intimate with because of everything they have shared and been through together.

It was with regular frequency that the women I spoke with talked about the importance of a lover who paid attention to their bodies and made them feel beautiful, sexy, and wanted. Carrie, 50 and recently divorced, said, "I've had two lovers in the last six months that have done more for me than many other things in my life. So that's been really healing." One of those lovers is a woman and the other is man. She was married for most of her adult life but realized that she is also attracted to women and is really enjoying the freedom to experiment sexually, and as she said, the experiences have done more for her body image than she could have imagined.

Several married women thought that it was easier to have a husband who is large or to have a husband who has shown that he is attracted to her regardless of her size: "I think body image wise—I guess in a selfish way, I think I have an easier time because my husband is fat, too. I don't know. Sometimes I just think in my mind, it might be hard if my husband was really thin. Maybe

I'd have lower self-esteem. The sex is fantastic. It's always funny to me, because it's hard to find plus-size maternity clothes. I think to myself, 'Gosh, do they think we don't have sex or something?' Or sexy clothes and stuff like that, but that's getting better" (Shawna, 34, white). Shawna has a great sex life with her husband, and when we spoke, baby number six was on the way. She mentioned that she has heard other women talk about discontinuing sex when they gain weight because they feel bad about their bodies. Her reaction to that is, "That's silly, because sex is one way to feel good about your body."

Age also seemed to help women become more comfortable sexually. It is not surprising that the older one gets, the more comfortable one becomes with her body. The women who were the youngest, under 25 or so, reported the most difficulty meeting partners, enjoying sex, and feeling confident undressing in the presence of a partner. Women in their late 30s and beyond were the most comfortable. Some of them directly attributed the change in their comfort levels to their age:

> As I've gotten older, I've been able to relax more in sex. Yeah, I've been able to relax more and enjoy sex and make it more about me and I think that's an age thing with just sex in general. When I was younger, I worried so much about "was I doing it right" and "am I sexy enough, am I doing this right, am I pleasing him, am I a good lay?" ... As I got older I started going, "Wait a minute. I didn't get mine." As I've gotten older I've been more concerned with getting mine and therefore just really enjoying the experience a lot more and worrying less about my body and about the enjoyment and I think that's just made all the difference in the world. (Mindy, 40, white)

Mindy's account of the difference between how she felt when she was young and how she feels now was common for many of the women. Even Krista, only 28, has noticed a change from her teen years and early twenties to her late twenties: "I think the clarity has kind of come from being older, because I was extremely worried about how other people perceived my weight when I was younger" (Krista, 28, white).

If fat is a threat to masculinity and femininity, then fat women who enjoy sex and set out to find partners are exceptionally subversive, because they are rejecting the conventional beauty messages and the gender-role norms that require women to wait for men to pursue them. This sort of thinking came from a number of women who are not feminist, or at least did not identify as feminist during the interview. As Jana so eloquently stated, "I think there's something threatening about a large woman who is confident, sexual, and powerful, because so much of the world is about trying to be perfect" (Jana, 45, white).

Many of these women thought their behaviors were transgressive, because most people do not expect women who are fat to have confidence or to like the way they look. There is so much pressure in Western cultures to look a certain way and meet the excruciatingly narrow beauty standards that it is practically heresy for a woman to be happy with her body—especially a fat woman. Women are taught to hate their bodies and that there is always something they can change or fix to improve their appearance (Wolf [1991] 2002). The dominant discourse suggests that people have control over their body shape and size either through hard work or through the consumption of goods and services. If we are not careful or critical, it is really easy to be influenced by the dominant ideology that we should all strive to look "perfect." So when a woman who is fat is happy with her looks and feels comfortable in her skin, we as a society are astonished because she is acting in a way that is not "normal" for women. Not only does she not fit the conventional beauty mandate; she is subversive because she likes the way she looks.

Embodiment of fat or improved body image helps women transgress the larger societal view that fat women are either nonsexual or hypersexual. For women of size, having a sexual lifestyle that is satisfactory is transgressive. It was not necessary for women to subscribe to size acceptance as long as they found other ways that they could change the reflection in the mirror (Gailey forthcoming). Frequently, it was not through weight loss or any other dramatic physical change at all—it was the way they thought about their body and their self-worth that needed to change. In fact, some of the women who had lost a significant amount of weight were fairly self-conscious because of excess skin and because they felt that when they lost weight that they became objectified, which they were generally not used to. Those who were able to change what they saw in the mirror seemed to find pleasure eating nutritious foods and exercising or getting some physical activity.

Conclusion

The dominant cultural discourse and framing of large bodies as unattractive serves as a form of social control that reinforces stereotypes and mistreatment of fat women. Messages stating that fat people (especially women) are lazy, gluttonous, lacking willpower, and nonsexual or hypersexual are repeated so frequently, and often without criticism, that many people assume they are true. The public also tends to believe that we have more control over our body size than we actually do. It is commonly assumed that fat women are at fault for any mistreatment they receive because they have chosen to remain fat and not lose weight.

Jessica wrote in an email to me after our interview,

> I also felt I should mention that as good as my self-image and self-confidence is now, I still lapse back into old patterns. I can be quite triggered if I feel sexually insecure; my husband has some health issues that can lessen his libido, and if he turns down my sexual advances, I can be very hurt and cry a lot and get angry and need a lot of reassurance that he still finds me attractive. That's also gotten better with time, and we've both learned to navigate that better, but I'm not sure if I'll ever get to a point where I'll never feel like that. But I'm also not that upset by that realization, either—I've come to see them as inevitable, but thankfully transient. (Jessica, 35, white)

Jessica has come a long way, but the relationship she is forging with her body is delicate. It is tremendously difficult to shift the messages that she has heard her whole life and to go against what the majority of the people in her culture believe. As a woman who is fat, she has been repeatedly reminded that she is unattractive and that her body is unsightly—overcoming that sort of conditioning demonstrates tremendous resolve.

The phenomenon of hyper(in)visibility locates fat women in a seemingly paradoxical position, because they are assumed to be either nonsexual or hypersexual. Participants talked about feeling like they were hyperinvisible when it came to attracting partners, having their sexual needs met, or having others recognize them as sexual. They spoke about hypervisibility when they noted that men would sometimes seek them out on Internet dating sites because of the assumption that fat women are desperate, easy, or pushovers. In addition, they also performed hypervisibility when they embodied fat hatred and expected and accepted mistreatment from partners. As I stated at the beginning of the chapter, the illusion of a paradox reinforces the status quo. Some of the women I talked with have transgressed the norms and are no longer allowing their self-worth, sexual satisfaction, or well-being to be dictated by the media and larger culture, even if they still have not fully come to terms with being fat. In the *Fat Studies* manuscript, I closed by stating that "the size acceptance movement has played a key role in helping these women resist patriarchal control by subverting the hegemonic view of women's bodies and their sexuality" (Gailey 2012, 126). It was so refreshing to talk with additional women who were not involved in size acceptance but still found ways to enjoy their body and sexuality.

Chapter 6

Embracing Fat Pride

It is incredibly difficult for the majority of women, regardless of their size, to embrace and accept their bodies. In fact, most women in the United States report that they are dissatisfied with their body and appearance (Bordo 1993; Hesse-Biber 2007). This dissatisfaction is so rampant that it has been dubbed "normative discontent" (Rodin, Silberstein, and Striegel-Moore 1985). Scholars have pointed to the unrealistic images of the female form in the media, the emphasis on dieting, the cornucopia of products designed to "fix" nearly any bodily flaw, the "obesity epidemic," and sundry other social conditions as the roots of normative discontent. As I discussed in Chapter 3, approximately half of the US population is on some sort of weight-loss diet at any given moment. The prevalence of normative discontent is so great in American culture that practically no one is immune. Research indicates that dissatisfaction with one's body appears in children as young as seven (Heron et al. 2013)—anecdotal evidence from students and friends who are parents indicates that age four is probably more accurate—and it is increasingly prevalent among elderly women (Lewis and Cachelin 2001).

Being attractive (thin)[1] carries with it a tremendous amount of privilege. Attractive people are frequently regarded as smarter, funnier, more capable, and nicer. Attractive (thin) persons earn more money than unattractive (fat) people and are more likely to be hired and promoted. Moreover, as a society we tend to hold the extreme belief that "what is beautiful is good." For instance, in a well-known social psychological study, participants were presented with a story about a little girl who throws a rock at a dog. In half of the stories, the girl was described as having an angelic appearance; in the other half, she was described as homely. When respondents were asked to indicate why the little girl threw the rock at the dog, those who read the story that featured an angelic-looking girl tended to attribute her actions to external causes: she must be having a bad day. On the other hand, those who read the story where the girl was described as homely tended to attribute her action to internal causes, such as being a bad girl (Dion 1972).

These findings are consistent with a plethora of research that shows that we tend to grant attractive (thin) people considerable leeway for their actions (Dion, Berscheid, and Walster 1972; Katz 2007; Rhode 2010; Wheeler and Kim 1997). Considering the benefits and privileges attached to thinness, it is no wonder that most of us aim to make ourselves "more attractive" by trying to lose weight or work hard to maintain our weight even if we are already thin. Attractive bodies have the privilege of being visible when it is important to be acknowledged while simultaneously remaining invisible when it comes to public scrutiny. Moreover, the hyper(in)visibility of fat bodies reminds us that there are serious social repercussions to having a fat (unattractive) body.

Laurie Ann Lepoff (1983) writes that she understands the privilege that comes with having a socially acceptable appearance firsthand. She reveals to her readers that for the first two years of high school, she was thin and her peers recognized her as smart. When she gained weight, she said that her peers' perception of her changed dramatically. They no longer believed she was smart and did not take her seriously. She writes that she was scorned and ridiculed (p. 204). She also experienced this same attitudinal shift later in life when she lost a lot of weight. She argues that the power and privilege that stems from being thin is invisible—it is an unmarked category. Unmarked categories obscure inequality, because those with privilege (the dominant group) are ignored and the focus is directed toward the subordinate group. For instance, when race issues are discussed, the assumption is that it concerns people of color, or if gender is discussed, the assumption is that the conversation is about women (Katz 1999; Saguy 2012).

I have shown throughout this book that there are women who transgress bodily norms by choosing to accept (or trying to accept) their body despite the incredible challenge of being a fat woman in a fatphobic society. A sizable proportion of this sample either (1) accepted their bodies (or were in the process of acceptance) but did not identify with the size acceptance movement or (2) embraced a fat identity through involvement (even minimal involvement) in the size acceptance movement.

In this chapter, I explore the size acceptance movement and the politics of a fat identity, embodiment of a fat identity, resistance strategies employed by the women who challenge the dominant framework of fat as unattractive and unhealthy, and the ways in which activists "do fat" in order to subvert the oppression of hyper(in)visibility. I also shed light on some of the limitations with the current size acceptance movement and difficulties some of the women I talked with experienced embodying a fat identity. In Western cultures, fat bodies are hyper(in)visible partially due to the cultural obsession with thinness and fear of fat. Considering that it is "normal" for "thin" or "average-sized" women to express dissatisfaction with their bodies and a desire to lose weight, it is, I think, even more remarkable that fat women are able to embrace their bodies and subvert the negative messages in a culture that is clearly obsessed with appearance.

SIZE ACCEPTANCE, NAAFA, AND THE POLITICS OF A FAT IDENTITY

The size acceptance movement began in the United States in 1969 when William Fabrey founded the National Association to Aid Fat Americans, which is now called the National Association to Advance Fat Acceptance (NAAFA). There have been numerous scholars and activists who have written extensively about the size acceptance movement, so I will not attempt that here.[2] In addition to NAAFA, there are smaller groups across North America, and even a few international groups, but none that compare with the size or influence of NAAFA.

In addition, there is an extensive online community—the "fat-o-sphere"—of people who identify as fat activists. They write blogs, tweet, participate in listservs devoted to the movement, engage in a plethora of social networking sites and pages, and are quite engaged in the scholarly research regarding fat, "obesity," and diseases commonly considered the result of "obesity." The goals of NAAFA and other size acceptance groups are not monolithic, but broadly speaking, all seek to (1) celebrate the diversity of body sizes and redefine what is considered an "acceptable body," (2) dismantle negative stereotypes associated with fat, and (3) end size discrimination.[3]

Fat acceptance activists challenge the medical and public health ideology that fat is unhealthy or unattractive. According to their alternative framework, fat is beautiful, healthy, a form of natural bodily diversity, and the basis for civil rights claims (Saguy 2013). Size acceptance advocates challenge the dominant frame by embracing the word *fat* as a basis of identity (recall from Chapter 2 that numerous women specifically did not want fat as part of their identity). *Fat* is a powerful word because it is most commonly used to injure or intimidate (thunder 1983). For instance, I have found that when I use *fat* to discuss my research, I must quickly preface it with an explanation and contextualization, because the audience becomes noticeably uncomfortable, which is not surprising; their discomfort reflects the pejorative nature of the word. Fat activists argue that reclaiming and embracing *fat* changes its effect, and that once reclaimed, it can no longer be used as a way to punish, humiliate, or hurt someone.

I should note that this position is not without controversy, even in the size acceptance community. In the April 2013 issue of NAAFA's newsletter, the organization indicated that they were considering changing the name of the organization. NAAFA stated, in part, that "with the pressure of society to demonize fat, organizations don't look at common goals and interests, and disregard NAAFA's requests for alliance because of our name. NAAFA needs to develop alliances and garner support of other organizations in order to further our goals in the civil rights and social justice arenas. We cannot continue to bury our heads in the sand and believe this problem will resolve itself. For us to effect change, we must be taken seriously."[4] This statement has been considered a divisive blow for some in the movement. There are those who support the idea of changing the name because the word *fat* is so deeply laden with negativity.[5] They argue that they have lost the battle trying to reclaim *fat* and need to shift to more inclusive descriptive terms, like *size acceptance* or *body acceptance*. One woman who supports the name change publicly stated on a forum that she does not hate her fat, but she does hate the word because of the way it was used against her as a child.

However, others on the forum noted how important it is to reclaim the word *fat* in their lives and how transformational that process has been. One woman posted that she is recovering from anorexia and that embracing *fat* has been instrumental to her recovery. She shared that before she found size acceptance, the word *fat* was terrifying to her because it meant that she was unlovable, unworthy, and disgusting, but now "it is simply an adjective that cannot and does not define who I am." She noted that if NAAFA changes the name to exclude *fat*, she would no longer support the organization.

Many who protested the name change cite the NAAFA Constitution, which states, "We choose to use the word *fat* to describe ourselves in order to remove the negative connotations normally associated with larger-than-average body size" (Article III, 2).[6] Those against the name change argue that removing *fat* from the name of the organization will further render fat persons unbeneficially invisible. Protestors noted that they "will not hide" and they will not allow NAAFA to hide them either.

One of the problems with the size acceptance movement is that it does not have a large, cohesive formal group like other social movements. The fat pride community tends to be based online and in books, and according to Saguy and Ward (2011, 69), this is the reason the movement has not developed a strong counterculture. This recent move by NAAFA to consider changing its name could further isolate the movement and divide its supporters, in turn making embracing fat pride even more difficult. Despite the fact that there are relatively few people involved in the movement in this sample, there are those who find community and strength online, and there were numerous women who credit the "fat-o-sphere" with helping them learn to embody a fat identity.

Being Seen and Embodying Fat

Depending on the social context, to be seen (visible) is either a form of acknowledgement or a form of critical observation. As I have demonstrated throughout the book, the women who spoke with me received tremendous scrutiny because of their body size, while they were simultaneously erased or ignored in situations that would benefit them socially. However, some of the women I talked with subvert the phenomenon of hyper(in)visibility by "coming out as fat" (Mitchell 2005; Saguy and Ward 2011; Sedgwick 2000).

In Chapter 2, I introduced the notion of coming out as fat as a way in which one begins to identify as a fat person. One comes out as fat by announcing to the world that she accepts her body and is no longer "living from the neck up." Such an act is empowering because it subverts the negativity surrounding fat when one begins to "own" or "embody" her fat rather than trying to change her body or lose weight. Some of the women rejected the idea of embodying a fat identity and preferred to live as women who "happen to be fat," whereas others noted that finding the size acceptance movement has helped them begin the arduous task of embodying their fat (see also Gailey 2012). Both are forms of embodiment, but there are qualitative distinctions.

The women who reject a fat identity but are committed to self-acceptance tend to see themselves as being more than their body. For instance, they felt that their genuine self (or who they are) is consistent and continuous, whereas their body might change. Some of them told me that when they were thin they were still smart, caring, conscientious, and funny. Many also noted that as they grow old and their bodies wrinkle and sag, their genuine self will still remain intact. Just because they have not, and likely will not, come out as fat does not mean they do not remain committed to the notion of self-love over self-hate. Moreover, they are working against the dominant norms of society that mandate that women be thin or be perpetually engaged in a battle to become thin (see also Gailey forthcoming).

Another important distinction between these two groups is that those who do accept their bodies but do not want a fat identity seem somewhat resigned to the fact that they are fat. They have reached a point where they know it is unlikely that their bodies will change or that they will lose weight. A commonly used phrase was "This is my body and I better get used to it." They have found that they can "get used" to their body, but they are not fat and proud, whereas the women who do identify with the fat acceptance movement seem to have embraced their fat (at least publicly). In this respect, they have come out as fat. As Charlotte Cooper (1998,

47) has said, "Coming out makes us visible, it shows that we are fine as we are. It is a personal step which has wider social and political consequences, such as the promotion of diversity."

The notion of coming out as fat is curious in one respect, because according to Goffman's (1963) typology, only those with invisible stigmas can pass as normal and come out, whereas fat is highly visible and readily apparent. Fat persons can cover—as we saw Cassie do in Chapter 2 when she tried to prevent her size from affecting her friends' dining experiences—but not pass. Saguy and Ward (2011) refine Goffman's concept of stigma in light of the fact that the size acceptance movement has appropriated the language of coming out. They reexamine the distinctions between coming out and flaunting. Flaunting is typically viewed as an instance where someone engages in a behavior that he or she is likely to be criticized for because of his or her stigmatized identity. For instance, a fat woman might be considered flaunting when she wears tight clothing, or a gay couple might be considered flaunting when they kiss in public.

Saguy and Ward (2011) found that the fat activists they interviewed discussed coming out and flaunting as happening simultaneously; flaunting fat provides an avenue for claiming inclusion. Along these lines, Marilyn Wann, a fat activist, said in an interview that when she orders vegetarian food or attends a yoga class, she is asserting her difference while simultaneously affirming her similarity in cultural tastes (Saguy and Ward 2011, 67).

However, the phenomenon of flaunting need not reflect the direct intentions of the flaunter. What may appear as flaunting may instead simply be a way of living one's life as a "normal" person. The gay couple who kisses in public or the fat woman who wears tight clothing are perceived as flaunting because they are marginalized and hyper(in)visible. From the perspective of the flaunters, they are simply engaging in behaviors that those who are socially unobtrusive engage in all the time without criticism.

Embodiment of a Fat Identity

The initial 36 women I interviewed for this book were all familiar with fat acceptance and NAAFA. Most were not NAAFA members, and the majority (63 percent) were not actively involved in the size acceptance movement. In other words, most were familiar with the movement because they read blogs, subscribed to listservs, and participated in various social networking sites, but they did not consider themselves activists. The following quote illustrates the typical involvement noted by the majority of the women in the first set of interviews: "Well, whenever they have a posting, like I get a digest of their stuff that's on Yahoo, and they don't have stuff every day that comes out. And they also don't post blogs daily on MySpace. So it's just intermittent. Whenever they send something out" (Janet, 36, white). Twenty-three women made statements similar to Janet's when I asked them how much time they spent on size acceptance activities. As is evident, most were passively involved.

Numerous women from the 2009 sample mentioned that they learned about size acceptance from Marilyn Wann's (1998) book *Fat!So?* In the book, Wann challenges the hegemonic views of fat and proclaims that no one should have to apologize for his or her size. Her book is full of wit, humor, advice, and anecdotes intended to reframe the view of fat. One interviewee stated that when she saw the book at the library she could not believe what she was reading and could not help thinking that Wann was asking the impossible. After several years of dieting unsuccessfully and continuous self-deprecation, she bought her own copy and is now committed to embracing a fat identity.

For some women, it took a major life event to lead them to challenge the views they had about their body and who they are as fat women:

> We divorced, bad, bad divorce. I actually had, it was almost my birth in the size acceptance movement I guess, up until that time I used to just consider myself, "Gosh, I'm a lucky fat woman that I have a family, that I have a professional job and things are wonderful." Then boom, things weren't wonderful. Anyway, one weekend he had the kids, I stripped down naked and walked around naked all weekend in my house and looked in mirrors and touched my body in ways I'd never touched it. Not sexual, just feeling it and thought, "You were that child, that adolescent, that young woman, that older woman, you're going to be fat the rest of your life. It's time to get used to it and move on." (Rita, 59, white)

Rita's weekend of "walking around naked" helped her learn to see her body differently and become accustomed to touching herself.

Rita's transformation started with what sounds like resignation—"you're going to be fat the rest of your life"—but she made it clear later in our conversation that she has adopted the principles of fat acceptance. For Rita, this exercise helped her connect her body to her genuine self and eliminate her internalized fatphobia. So many women that I talked with tried to ignore or forget their bodies by not looking at their body (below the neck) in the mirror and by not touching themselves. Rita was "born into the size acceptance movement" through the realization that she must overcome her body hatred so that she could progress and renew.

The choice to renew and reinterpret oneself more positively takes commitment, perseverance, and will. As thunder (1983, 212, emphasis in original) writes in her chapter featured in *Shadow on a Tightrope*, "Going from *being* a fat woman *to coming out* as a fat woman is not an easy journey to plot . . . it's more gradual evolution than sudden change." I heard this message repeated from the women I spoke with, too. Moreover, it was common for women to note that there is an internal struggle between their public and private selves:

> I am right now [accepting of self] but I have major moments where I hate the fat. I hate looking like this. I hate being fat. It's easier to be self-accepting when talking to someone about it in any general sense, you, my best friend. The first time my best friend saw me have a major breakdown about being fat and a lot of it was always very connected to the fact that I didn't really have any real relationships until basically my husband. I had that one with the married guy, but that lasted four months. I had never had any relationship more than six months. I only dated three guys, actually dated. Most of it [the breakdown] was related to not being in a relationship. That I was never going to meet anyone. No one could deal with me being fat, blah, blah, blah, blah, blah. The first time that she saw me have a breakdown when it came to being fat she just was like, "What is this? This is not you." I'm like "I have them just like everyone else." I don't know what will always trigger it. Sometimes it's in my own head. Sometimes it's whatever somebody else says. (Elizabeth, 30, white)

Elizabeth is conflicted. Sometimes the destructive messages are too overwhelming and she has difficulty accepting herself. It was fairly common for the women who said they embody a fat identity to tell me that they struggle with acceptance privately but that publicly they would never let on. Many of those who told me that they have come out still seem to vacillate between resignation and affirmatively embracing their bodies:

> You know, I'm really happy with how I am physically. I struggle with fat hatred still anyway. You know, like internalized fat hatred, shame—it's a paradox. I thought at this point it would diminish. I mean it's certainly diminished. It's not like I live with daily anxiety or self-hatred, or like—and I certainly never entertain seriously the thought that I need to change my body in any way, because I don't. But it's still—it's a struggle. It's a struggle. It can be a struggle to not hate myself for being a fat person. And—I mean, in a lot of ways I experience it now, I'm sort of like I look at myself, I realize that I'm very fat, and I'm like do I have to hate myself for that? And like, you know, I can't. I just can't. I can't. (Mary, 40, white)

Mary, like Elizabeth, notes that she is more accepting than not, but it is hard to silence the internalized fat hatred and to disregard the fat hatred propagated throughout the culture. It might be even more difficult for some because of the lack of a "fat community." There is the virtual community, but most of the women I spoke with did not have Big Beautiful Women (BBW) groups or other fat accepting groups in their local area. The majority of the women were completely isolated from real, personal interaction with others from their community: "And I feel weird because I'm telling myself I'm beautiful, my body is lovely, it's almost like there is this second voice underneath it that is saying—that sort of is repeating all of the cultural messages that your body is ugly, that you are gluttonous and a slob and unlovable, and so it's like two different messages and I think what I try and do is make the positive voice just a little bit louder and drown out the other voice, and that is sort of how I see the world looks at your body" (Abigail, 23, white). Both Mary and Abigail struggle to silence the negative messages. However, they and numerous other women indicated that it does become easier with practice, and this is why the community of size acceptance is crucial, even if it is mostly online. When they start to feel badly about themselves, they can easily access others who sympathize and who are actively posting fat positive pictures, writing fat positive stories, and fact-checking media reports about the harms of fat. What is most impressive and promising is that most of these women are not activists and are minimally involved in the size acceptance movement, but they still reap the rewards of community engagement.

Embodiment of a discredited identity is no easy feat (Goffman 1963). The women who have begun to identify with the size acceptance's ideology are beginning to overcome the self-loathing and hatred that they have dealt with for years, but it is an extremely trying process. At one moment, they embody their fat and are working toward self-acceptance, yet at another, they struggle with the cultural messages and social forces that reinforce the hegemonic view that fat is unhealthy, unattractive, and something to lose at all costs. Fatphobia is entrenched in the discourse and institutionalized within North American culture. As many of the women stated, they are torn between two contradictory messages (I discuss the difficulties with embodying fat later in the chapter). It became apparent from the interviewees that activism and resistance, even the most passive forms of activism, strengthened embodiment.

It is important to note that there were 5 women from the 2009 sample who identified as activists, and their stories, while similar, do not represent the experience of the majority of the women. In the second set of interviews from 2012, I talked with 38 women, and only 2 of them fully adopted the size acceptance ideology, and none were activists.

When I asked women in the second set of interviews if they had ever heard of size acceptance, seven women responded with conviction that fat acceptance is an excuse or a rationalization. They almost all stressed that it was an example of people trying to say, "They're OK, but they're not OK. It can't be how they really feel" (Elaine, 52, white). Aisha similarly stated, "I don't think there's such a thing as anybody being happy being overweight. I hear people say that, I'm happy with my size. I'm happy the way I am. I love my body. That's rubbish. We all said that. I said that. It's not true" (Aisha, 31, African). Elaine, Aisha, and several others made it clear that they thought it was impossible to be fat and happy or fat and proud. However, it was apparent from some of the women I spoke with and from my observations of size acceptance groups, listservs, and forums that there are those who are fat and proud and who resist embodying a "spoiled identity," so there remains hope that others can also benefit from the message of body acceptance.

Refracting the View

Resistance to a stigmatized identity can come in multiple forms, but one of the ways that people cope with adversity is to connect with others who are similarly stigmatized (Goffman 1963). Size acceptance groups serve as a way to counter a deviant identity (Farrell 2011) by providing members with a vehicle to resist fat hatred and shame. One woman stated,

> I think I probably helped other people out that are, you know, maybe less secure than I am, that are maybe just discovering this idea that maybe there's nothing wrong with you if you're heavy. And it's just something that I feel like I need to monitor, because there are some very disturbing things happening. Sort of—just in the way that medical research is reported in the press, and the way that fat people are being blamed for the deficiencies of medical systems, both in the U.S. and other places. I think they're being scapegoated. I just think that there's—it's kind of dangerous what's going on, and that, you know, intelligent people who are willing to do something about it need to keep an eye on it and keep talking about it. (Lisa, 39, white)

Lisa thinks that the attention on the "obesity epidemic" is dangerous because it fuels fat hatred and bullying, or in other words, it perpetuates the phenomenon of hyper(in)visibility. Size acceptance groups and resources counter some of the negativity and provide group members with a "safe space," a sense of identity, and a place where they feel they belong:

> I think the most important thing to come out of this will be a sense of identity. That maybe we can—even if we don't get the laws changed, even if we don't have this huge social movement where everybody is OK with fat, and everybody believes that fat is—it's all right; you can be healthy if you're fat, even if none of that stuff ever happens, that it will give a sense of identity to people and a sense of privacy to other people. That they will understand that just because it's not how you want to live, and just because it's not what you think is necessarily correct, that it's an option, and it's not your place to say otherwise. And that's what I hope really comes out of it. That, you know, you teach your kids that everyone is equal. (Karen, 24, white)

For numerous women, the importance of the virtual community of size acceptance has changed their lives, especially in the absence of an in-person size acceptance community. These women talked with me about the importance of reading positive messages about fat or seeing fat bodies engaged in "normal" activities:

> Well, just any—any tool that you can have that makes you feel better about yourself, I think that's just immeasurably good. Just to get to the point where I'm not—where I don't feel like I have to be apologetic to people, just you know, you hear a positive message long enough, and it starts to impact you. For instance, I wouldn't go swimming in the summertime, because who wants to see me in a swimsuit? But then I realized—hearing this positive message online over and over, I'm like well, my daughter wants to go swimming, you know? It's either I put myself in a bathing suit and I take her swimming, or she doesn't go swimming. And then it's—and then she's 15, and she's complaining to her friends that my mom would never take me swimming as a kid. I don't know how to swim. You know, so it's just encouraging me to live my life now and stop putting things off until I magically become thin. (Carol, 30, white)

Through her limited exposure to size acceptance via the Internet, Carol has stopped waiting to become thin and has decided to start living her life as a fat woman.

Research has shown that genetics play a larger role in one's body size than is commonly accepted (see Bouchard et al. 1990). The burden of the stigma and self-hate began to disappear for Carol, Lisa, and others and when they realized what they intuitively already knew: that much of the information propagated by the media, politicians, and "health advocates" about the choice and irresponsibility of fat is erroneous or, for the most part, blown out of proportion (see Campos 2004 for a review). Another woman told me that she struggled for years trying to understand why she was fat when she ate the same amount of food as other nonfat people. With the help of the size acceptance movement, she has discovered that she is fat not because she is gluttonous, lazy, or an overeater; she is fat because she is a larger person: "I'm not an overeater. I eat normally and I'm fat. It's always been that way from the time I've been a little girl. And I thought this is ridiculous. I'm just going to let my body become the size it's going to be, because

I'm sick of this. I'm healthy. I'm active. There is no reason for not being that way" (Beth, 60, white). Not everyone who is fat is fat because they have a genetic predisposition, but there are many people for whom genetics is the contributing factor in their size, and for them, keeping weight off over the long term is unlikely and potentially harmful (Berg 1999; Campos et al. 2006; Cogan 1999; Garner and Wooley 1991). The majority of the 74 women have been fat since childhood. There were some who discussed overeating and even binge eating, as discussed in Chapter 3, but most thought that they had dieted themselves to their current weight or were genetically predisposed. The point here is that the size acceptance movement has provided those across a diverse range of contexts who are also willing to embrace the movement with the tools to combat the negative messages and misinformation. While the clear majority were not activists, it was the activists, online or otherwise, who helped lead them to personal change and the embodiment of fat.

Doing Fat as Activism

Charlotte Cooper (2009, as cited in Saguy and Ward 2011, 68) explains, "Somehow, embracing fat stereotypes enabled us to subvert them, and perhaps rob them of their power over us." Previously, I have discussed doing fat as one of the ways that hyper(in)visibility is perpetuated and reinforced. But what Cooper and other activists suggest is publicly subverting hyper(in)visibility to bring attention to fat oppression.

Through art, performance, comedy, and protest, some fat activists attempt to shift the collective view of fat as deviant or abhorrent. They seek to normalize the fat body by engaging in behaviors that many fat persons avoid publicly, like eating, exercising, or going swimming. The Adipositivity Project is a website created by fat activist photographer Substantia Jones. Her website features photos of nude or seminude fat women engaged in activities that are typically reserved for thin women. Her site is devoted to presenting adiposity in a positive light by photographing fat bodies. One of the photographs, which received a lot of attention because it was stolen from the site and used as a fat-shaming tool, is a picture of a fat woman in a bikini walking in the rain on the streets of New York. The "comedian" who stole the photograph used it to make fun of fat women, but the intent of Jones was to demonstrate the beauty and ordinariness of fat.

Fatphobia perpetuates hyper(in)visibility, but flaunting or coming out as fat can shift hyper(in)visibility (see also Saguy and Ward 2011). Engaging in public events such as smashing scales, bikini swim meets, and ice cream eat-ins redefines the way the public views fat. Marilyn Wann organized a public protest outside a local gym that had sponsored a billboard stating that fat people were in mortal danger because when the space aliens arrived they would eat fat people first. Wann and other fat activists engaged in aerobics outside the gym while holding signs that read, "I'm Yummy" or "Bite my Fat Alien Butt" (Saguy 2013, 155–56). These are wonderfully whimsical and effective ways to subvert the typical way fat bodies are encountered and publicly seen.

Whimsy and kitschy demonstrations queer fat body politics through resistance to the essentialist framing of fat as revolting and unchangeable. As LeBesco (2001, 83, emphasis in original) states, "We can begin to envision *fat play*, rather than *fat pathology*." She argues for an antiessentialist position of a fat identity that rejects causal explanations of fatness and instead focuses on the ways individuals create corporeal meaning materially and symbolically.

Mitchell (2005), a Canadian fat activist, writes about a group she cofounded called Pretty Porky and Pissed Off. The group has engaged in numerous demonstrations that transgress the dominant view of fat women. They engage in what they call "fat drag." Mitchell describes fat drag as similar to how drag queens perform femininity. They parody and exaggerate the beliefs about fat. For instance, four of the original members of Pretty Porky and Pissed Off have performed on multiple occasions a choreographed routine to "Baby Elephant Walk" by Henry Mancini wearing leotards and each carrying a birthday cake. They place the cakes on chairs while they dance and accentuate their bodies, especially the largest parts of their bodies, and for the finale they each sit on a cake, smashing it with their "big fat butts." Mitchell says that the cake dance is all about "having our cake and eating it too" (Mitchell 2005, 220).

Pretty Porky and Pissed Off has also engaged in street demonstrations. In 1996, they gathered on Queen Street, a popular shopping district for club wear in Toronto. They all wore tight-fitting outfits with loud colors, prints, and feather boas. The signs that they carried read "FAT!" and were printed on plastic picnic tablecloths (Mitchell 2005, 217). They gave away candy and information about the average size of North American women (size 12). Some of the demonstrators approached Sunday shoppers and asked, "Do you think I'm fat?" Mitchell describes the event as stripping away the power of the word *fat*. They took the phenomenon of hyper(in)visibility and usurped its power. They were hypervisible, but they were in control and used that hypervisibility to point out the manner in which fat women are rendered invisible (by the clothing stores on the street that did not carry plus sizes). According to Mitchell (2005), the Sunday shoppers were caught off guard or did not know how to respond to the fact that these fat women were flaunting their bodies and calling themselves fat.

Several of the women I spoke with who identified as activists also engaged in performances that subverted and transgressed fat: "So far, right now, my art is my vehicle for my fat activist ideas and my paintings show—I don't know—revolve around using images of large bodies and particularly my own, and inserting women into landscapes and trying to play with people's perceptions and ideas about fat bodies and trying to like turn it around a little bit, offer something new" (Pam, 29, white). Pam's art represents a transgression of the phenomenon of hyper(in)visibility. Rather than fat existing in a realm where it is Othered and marginalized, Pam's art attempts to redefine our view of fat by representing fat as "normal," beautiful, and art worthy.

Brenda Oelbaum, a fat activist and artist, uses her art to chronicle her dieting experiences. In a nine-minute video, she literally eats the pages of a diet book to demonstrate how mundane, banal, monotonous, and tasteless diets are.[7] Brenda was not always an activist. She spent the majority of her life, beginning at age 12, dieting and trying to lose weight. Along the way, she reportedly suffered anorexia and bulimia. As with so many others, every time she lost weight, she regained it and sometimes more. Brenda has quit dieting and eats what she wants, which she says has led her to stop obsessing about food. She also uses her art as a way to challenge and subvert the diet industry and the notion that fat is unattractive.

Tina, upon finding the size acceptance movement, began publicly speaking and performing fat in a manner that countered the stereotypes. I asked her why, and she said because no one else was doing it. She told me that her most recent form of activism involved writing a one-woman show: "I wrote a one-woman show on the fat ladies of the circus, and I perform that and talk about discrimination and assumptions, both the historical and current. Later this year, I'm hoping to start going into schools with it" (Tina, 34, white).

Beth, 60 and white, told me stories about her days of fat activism in the 1980s and 1990s. She and others from a local chapter of NAAFA in California had booths at "body expos" and passed out pencils or pens that read "fat chicks rule" or "fat power," and they talked with people about body image. They also attended informational meetings about weight-loss surgery and would ask the presenters extraordinarily difficult questions to call attention to the fact that there was not a lot of scientific evidence backing up the safety or even effectiveness of weight-loss procedures. She noted that they frequently were escorted out and had to stop because they feared arrest. Moreover, she told me that they used to hold demonstrations in a large public park on "International No Diet Day" and smash scales, pass out posters that said "no diet zone," and give out bracelets that read "love your body." They also put bookmarks that read "accept your body" in fashion magazines and diet books at a local Barnes & Noble.

Doing fat as activism involves engaging in behaviors that fat women are typically excluded from or told they should not engage in publicly. They parody the stereotypes of fat to point out the problems inherent in discrimination and fat shaming. Their goals are to challenge and subvert the taken-for-granted assumptions the public holds about fat women and their place in society. Fat activists proclaim to the world that they will not be rendered hyperinvisible or forced into the seclusion of their homes to feel sorry for themselves. Instead, they come out proud.

Some Concerns about Reinforcing the Dominant Frame through Fat Pride

A question one is bound to ask when thinking through the spectrum of choices, struggles, and achievements fat women face in the predicament of hyper(in)visibility is, how does a woman who is fat in a fatphobic society come to a point where she simply changes her mind about the way she sees her body? As we have seen, the embodiment of a fat identity is a complicated process. In *The Fat Female Body*, Samantha Murray (2008) raises some concerns with the embodiment of a fat identity and the size acceptance movement. For example, she argues that fat activists rely too heavily on "humanist logic of the primacy of the individual and the power of *rationality* in *overcoming* one's lived reality" (p. 108, emphasis in original). The process of coming out fat rests on the assumption that there is a gap between the mind and the body. In other words, it presumes a person can simply change her mind about her body. Someone who has a stigma that is invisible, like homosexuality, can come out without having to privilege her mind over her body because she can pass as "normal." When someone who is gay comes out, he or she is revealing something about himself or herself that was previously unknown (unseen). But a person who is fat—whose stigma is highly visible—must announce to the world that she *knows* she is fat but that she is *accepting of her fat* and not trying to lose weight or waiting to become thin. Unlike the person with the invisible stigma, the person with a hypervisible stigma must overcome the way she *sees* her body.

In addition, the process of embodying one's fat implies that fat is an empirical fact rather than a social construct. For instance, in the United States, one is "obese" (fat) when she has a body mass index (BMI) of 30 or greater, but not if she has a BMI of 28. In Taiwan, one is "obese" when she has a BMI of 27, but not 26. Does this mean that if my BMI is 28, I am not fat in the United States but I am fat in Taiwan? And recall that these categories are not static. Prior to June 17, 1998, a BMI of 30 was "overweight" because the "obese" cutoff was 32, but the categories shifted and the following day a BMI of 30 was considered "obese." In essence, how and who we label fat or "obese" are socially constructed and vary across time and culture. The size acceptance movement's suggestion that one embrace one's fat seems to reinforce the idea that fat is an empirical reality and downplay fat as a social construction (Murray 2008).

Another potential concern with the size acceptance movement for some of the interviewees involves what seems to be replacing one body standard with another ideal form. Nicole, a graduate student who has an academic and personal interest in Fat Studies and the size acceptance movement, told me that she was struggling with some guilt—actually she started crying when the topic came up—because she was in the process of beginning an exercise routine and was also trying to eat more healthfully (she defined it as cutting back on fast food). She had lost a little weight and felt really great about it, for the most part. When she started crying, I asked her what was wrong, and she told me that she felt like she was betraying the size acceptance movement because she was losing weight, especially because she was happy about it. She was conflicted because the little bit of weight she had lost and the increase in activity and healthier eating was making her feel better. She noted that she was not as winded when she took the stairs and was feeling better in general. But the fact that she felt better and was inspired to lose weight made her feel like she was turning her back on the size acceptance movement—she said she felt like a traitor.

Similarly, Cassie, 33 and white, had had weight-loss surgery because her weight was causing her serious mobility problems—to the point she where could not take care of herself—but she felt horrible about having the surgery. She knew she needed to do something drastic so that she could live without someone else having to clean and care for her, but she felt that by having weight-loss surgery she was betraying her sisters in the movement. She blogged about her feelings and found that she had tremendous support, but when we spoke about it she was still unsure. Weight-loss surgery contradicted everything she believed in, and she said she was angry with herself for having to have it.

Some of the other women reconciled feelings of guilt by discussing the Health at Every Size (HAES)® principles of "healthier eating" and exercise. Some of them, not all, lost a little weight when they began to employ HAES® and did not feel guilty about it because HAES® is readily accepted by the movement. It is disconcerting if supporters—that is, those who are trying to accept their bodies by following the writings of the size acceptance movement—feel guilty or shameful when they lose weight. It appears as if some adherents (or onlookers) believe that the size acceptance movement is reinforcing or advocating for a particular (or correct) body paradigm—one that is fat rather than thin.

As Murray (2008, 110) argues, "Not only is the 'fat' body being (re)valued over the normatively 'thin' body, but the mind is being privileged over the body." The insistence that one can simply abandon all the cultural knowledge about fat and ignore the dominant discourse and systems of power is an ideology that many social theorists, such as Judith Butler, argue against. Moreover, it plays into the medical model—that activists' themselves challenge—that assumes that the body is something that can be treated, fixed, and altered as if it were separate from the person with the "condition."

However, I am not arguing that the size acceptance movement is not helpful or fails to provide a welcome and necessary resource, because the evidence I have presented in this book and published previously indicates that it is (see Gailey 2012). I and others, such as Murray, fear that the message is a bit too simplistic, which is the reason some women who passionately want and choose to embody size acceptance feel guilty when they try to lose weight or even lose weight unexpectedly, as one woman did when she was put on a stimulant after being diagnosed with attention deficit disorder. Recall that the majority of participants indicated that they are torn between two contradictory messages. Privately those who embodied a fat identity (not the five activists) found themselves wanting to lose weight and would even "take the magic pill" if it were offered, but publicly they put forth a strong and confident outlook.

One of the major limitations with doing fat as a form of activism and transgression is that it may have the effect of reinforcing the dominant views of fat. For instance, BBW groups, bikini swim parties, negligée parties, beauty contests, fashion shows, and so forth all send the message that a woman's value is in her body and appearance, which is tied to patriarchy and heteronormativity, so rather than challenging and critiquing these institutions, it plays directly into them. Fat women are excluded from the privilege that comes with having a thin body and so they, too, want to engage in the activities that thin women do, but these behaviors are far from radical. Some of the women I interviewed in 2009 told me that they were not members of NAAFA because they felt like many of the activities reinforced heteronormativity and the male gaze. Several others noted that they did not feel that they were accepted at NAAFA events because they were "not fat enough." In fact, it was mentioned to me on numerous occasions that those at the smaller end of the fat spectrum are often treated as outsiders at NAAFA events.

In her blog "Fat Enough to Belong,"[8] Sally E. Smith asks, "Who is fat enough to belong in size acceptance?" She asks this question not because she wants to create guidelines for who can and cannot benefit from the size acceptance movement but because there are tensions among those who are at the highest end of the weight spectrum and those who are "midsize fat" or "small fat" (i.e., "inbetweenies").[9] This tension is largely about privilege. In contemporary society, "smaller fat" people are deemed more "acceptable" than larger fat or supersize fat persons. The concern for some involved in NAAFA or similar size acceptance organizations is that "inbetweenies" are unaware of their unearned privilege (just as many white people are unaware of their unearned privilege in US society).

Moreover, on fat fashion blogs, smaller fat women tend to receive more compliments and comments than larger fat women. According to Smith's blog, there have been cases where some small fat people avoided inviting supersized fat people to events or outings because they "did not want to deal with the special needs of the larger person." These sorts of occurrences can create friction in the size acceptance community about "who belongs." This is not unique to the size acceptance movement. Other social movements have experienced intragroup tensions based on perceived opportunities and privileges. As Smith aptly notes, "We can't seem to escape perpetuating and reinforcing the oppression we face."[10] Smith reminds readers that size acceptance is not just for those who are the fattest; rather, it is for everyone.

The dominant framework that fat is unhealthy, ugly, and symbolic of excess is institutionalized within American culture, which is why attempting social change through individuals is unlikely to promote change in society. It might behoove size activists to attempt to place an emphasis on fat as a social construction and impact change on a structural level, rather than only on an individual level (I discuss this more in Chapter 7). This is not to say that activists should not engage in hypervisible activities. As Murray (2008) argues, the movement might consider that its current message—that one should love their fat body—ignores the larger reality that this task is tremendously difficult in the current social structure.

Conclusion

In this chapter, I demonstrated the qualitative distinctions between those who accept their body but deny a fat identity and those who embrace a fat identity. The latter have come out to tell the world that they will no longer allow themselves to feel ashamed, less than, or Othered. The former, also briefly discussed at the end of Chapter 2, seem to have reached a point of resignation about their body but do not want their identity wrapped up in their body—they are accepting but not embracing.

I also discussed the size acceptance movement, NAAFA, and the politics of a fat identity. There are tensions within NAAFA regarding the use of the word *fat*. NAAFA is considering changing its name because the word *fat* is so laden with pejorative baggage. The leaders of the organization hope that by changing the name they will attract more members, greater public acceptance, and corporate sponsorship. Those opposed to the name change argue that changing the name is "selling out" and rendering fat people invisible. The fact that NAAFA is even considering changing its name points to the pervasiveness of the phenomenon of hyper(in)visibility. If the oldest and largest organization fighting for fat persons' rights and civil liberties feels it has to hide from the word *fat*, how will the discrimination against fat persons and the propagation of misinformation about fat ever stop?

These interviews revealed that those who have come to a point where they are no longer simply resigning to the fact that they are fat, but instead are embracing their fat and are ready to literally and symbolically tell the world that they accept and embrace their body, sometimes struggle with how to put that into practice. For instance, some of the women noted that they frequently have to silence their internal negativity about their body or fat in general.

They want to embrace a fat identity, but they vacillate between embodiment and feelings of resignation. Many noted that when they are feeling down, the "fat-o-sphere" helps pick them up and make them feel better about their body and self.

Fat activists subvert the phenomenon of hyper(in)visibility by doing fat. Some, like members of Pretty Porky and Pissed Off, engage in behaviors that parody and exaggerate the public's perception of fat women. They make themselves visible—even hypervisible—on their own terms. Other fat activists hold public events such as smashing scales, outdoor group aerobics, or ice cream eat-ins to challenge the stereotypes that fat women are self-loathing, passive, and always on a diet.

Unfortunately, the push toward embodiment of a fat identity by fat activists is incredibly challenging to enact. Several women who were working hard to embody their fat selves and take on a fat identity admitted that they struggled privately with the notion of fat acceptance. In fact, they almost always accepted their body, but their message connoted more resignation than celebration. Others admitted that they felt guilty when they have lost weight, because they felt like they were betraying the movement. This is problematic, because size acceptance is, or at least ought to be, about self-acceptance no matter one's size, shape, or weight.

Moreover, Murray (2005, 2008) argues that the process of coming out fat assumes that there is a mind/body split. For instance, it requires that one be able to rationally overcome her lived reality and assumes that fat is an empirical fact rather than a social construction. This is easier said than done. The institutionalization of fat hatred and the seemingly unending messages that are propagated by the media and others about the dangers of fat and how unattractive fat bodies are makes it terribly difficult to be "rational" about one's body. The embodiment of a fat identity is complex and emotional. It requires tremendous commitment, perseverance, determination, and will.

On August 26, 2013, Michel Martin, host of NPR's "Tell Me More," told listeners that the show's executive producer, Teshima Walker Izrael, died from colon cancer. In remembrance, Michel played a clip of Teshima talking about her experiences as a fat Black woman. When I heard Teshima speak about the complexities of embodying fat in a fatphobic and racist culture, I knew I had to discuss it in this chapter. Teshima's voice beautifully and articulately brought to life the challenges that were communicated to me by so many of the women I interviewed. Teshima begs for roles that depict *real* fat Black women, ones whose lives are complicated and nuanced. For instance, she says, "I'd have modest fat girls and juicy, fat vixens that wear tight, short skirts with 5-inch heels. I'd have fat, evil executives that shout at everyone to hell, and I'd have the lovable fat woman that had two men vying for her attention."[11]

Teshima's statement embodies the ways in which fat women, specifically fat Black women, are rendered invisible or hyperinvisible through one-dimensional characters and clichéd stereotypes in film and television. She asks producers to have the courage to create fat women characters who are complex and nuanced, just as thin characters are. She admits that there are times when she struggles to accept her body and tells listeners that she, too, sometimes considers diet pills, personal trainers, and even weight-loss surgery. When she says, "I want to be healthy," I take it to mean that she wants to accept her body and treat herself well, not starve or overexercise or try to force her body into a shape that is not her.

Teshima and the women I interviewed wish for something more from popular culture and the average stranger. They want to be seen as people, not spectacles, and to be treated with dignity and respect. While many of these women still struggle with being fat, for the most part, the women I discussed in this chapter are making strides toward self-acceptance.

Chapter 7

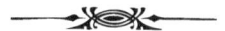

Shifting the Focus

Subverting the Judgmental Gaze: Why These Stories Matter

When the research for this project concluded and I decided to write a book, rather than publish a series of journal articles, one of my goals was to give voice to the amazing women who shared their time and stories with me. As I listened to, read, and reread the transcripts of these interviews, the overarching theme that came through was the phenomenon of hyper(in)visibility. The women I interviewed talked about their identities, dieting histories, health, sexual and relationship experiences, and the way they are treated and perceived by the larger culture within the spectrum of visibility. They recounted instances where they felt they were made into a spectacle while shopping in the grocery store, at the gym, or in the doctor's office. Some of the women told harrowing stories of near-death experiences because physicians failed to see past their body size, or they recounted instances where intimate partners took advantage of them because their needs were not viewed as "important," while others described occasions where family members denigrated them, neglected them, and overlooked their pain and humiliation. But these women also made it clear that they are incredibly strong, resilient, and perseverant despite the predicament of hyper(in)visibility and sordid typecasts.

The stereotypes associated with fat women are pervasive and harmful to all of us. In *Black Feminist Thought*, Patricia Hill Collins (1990) argues that the stereotypes of Black women (as the Mammy or temptress) work as "controlling images" that serve to reinforce the hegemonic viewpoint for everyone, including

African American women. In other words, stereotypes of marginalized groups perpetuate power for those in privileged and dominant positions. The blame is then shifted to those who are marginalized rather than to the social structures responsible for their oppression. Collins argues that if marginalized groups are given a voice, or if their stories are told from their standpoint, those who are oppressed can gain power, control, and knowledge over their own lives. In essence, she argues that as those who are oppressed become occupants of a standpoint, they also become knowing subjects in their own right, rather than merely objects that are known by others. This is one of the reasons why I set out to collect the stories of women of size and why this book makes an important contribution both academically and, perhaps more important, socially.

These "controlling images" (Collins 1990) of the gluttonous, lazy, unhealthy, unkempt, or unattractive fat woman harm all women (and men), because we become afraid of being/getting/becoming fat. We can all see the tremendous scrutiny that women who are fat are under, and we become "docile bodies" (Foucault 1977), policing and disciplining ourselves for fear that someone is watching and will punish us for not meeting the prescribed standards for being a "normal" woman.[1]

In this final chapter, I return to a discussion of fatphobia and the "obesity epidemic." I also focus on the heuristic and academic importance of the concept of hyper(in)visibility for discussing marginalized bodies. The concept has broad application and illustrates how interactions and societal messages reinforce and perpetuate inequality and Othering. I close with some modest suggestions for shifting the focus away from body weight to an emphasis on the appreciation of the diversity of human bodies and offer insights regarding how to subvert the hegemonic discourse.

Fatphobia and the War on "Obesity"

The data collected from these interviews demonstrates that these women are not a monolithic group with one lived experience, nor do they share a uniform point of view about what it means to be a fat woman in contemporary society. Some of the women were extremely dissatisfied with their appearance and were working hard to lose weight, whereas others were invested in bodily acceptance. Some reported good health, whereas others had serious concerns (with or without actual problems). For instance, a number of the women had minor health problems such as hypothyroidism, polycystic ovarian syndrome, or diabetes, and a few even had life-threatening illnesses or debilitating ailments such as cancer or lipedema. Several women discussed histories of abuse and degradation by partners, whereas others reported overwhelmingly positive experiences and loving relationships. Not surprisingly, those with health problems and the least positive sexual experiences tended to be more invested in losing weight and rejecting a fat identity. In contrast, the women with good health or only a few health concerns and who enjoyed more positive sexual and relationship experiences tended to be committed to self- and bodily acceptance. Of those in the latter group, a few even embraced a fat identity.

However, what they all have in common is the burden of negotiating a culture that is extraordinarily fatphobic. Until I began studying this topic, I had no idea how omnipresent fatphobia is in society. Amanda Levitt, the founder of the website "Bodypositive .com," told a *USA Today* reporter that she receives a copious amount of hate mail with messages like "Go be fat somewhere else," "You're going to die ugly," and "Shame on you and your disgusting bodies."[2] Levitt said that most of the mail contains vulgarity, and some writers have gone so far as to suggest Levitt should commit suicide. Unfortunately, this sort of unconstructive opining and vilification are all too common on blog posts or other articles that are "fat positive" (in addition to everyday lived experiences). Several of the women I talked with who frequently blog told me that Internet "trolls" post these types of comments on their blogs regularly (I immediately started reading the comments on blogs and fat positive articles and found this to be true). For instance, some Fat Studies books have received scathing "reviews" on Amazon that have little to do with the content of the book.

Abigail Saguy's (2013) book *What's Wrong with Fat* received at least one "review" in which the "reviewer" clearly had neither read the book nor taken a moment to review Saguy's scholarly credentials; this person wrote "more fat logic from a fat person" and went on to claim that "99.9 percent of obese people are fat because they EAT TOO MUCH bad food." This "reviewer" also said that Professor Saguy is "intellectually and factually challenged and NOTHING she says or writes is even remotely supported by facts, data or science." Amy Farrell's book (2009) *Fat Shame* has also received several hateful and disrespectful "reviews" that are overly ripe with misinformation about fat. The comments of these "reviewers" shine light on the fact that "obesity" and fat are extraordinarily touchy subjects in which some people are surprisingly committed to spewing hateful and misleading information. I share these examples because they are indicative of what happens when the hegemonic view of fat is challenged and they demonstrate how tightly fat hatred is woven into the cultural fabric.

As I was writing this chapter, Ragen Chastain, author of the blog *Dances with Fat*, wrote a piece about "normalizing obesity"—the claim that anyone who does not portray fat people as miserable or in other stereotypical terms is accused of "normalizing obesity." Regan wrote, "Any media outlet, television show, movie etc. that shows fat people being successful at anything other than weight loss will be immediately criticized for normalizing obesity."[3] Having a fat body, writing about size acceptance, or even suggesting that people of size deserve respect, dignity, and equal treatment under the law frequently leads to vitriolic outbursts and the perpetuation of the phenomenon of hyper(in)visibility.

One of the frequent questions I am asked when I present this research or discuss it in public is, "Aren't you worried about promoting unhealthy lifestyles?" My response to this question is twofold. First, as a sociologist I am interested in understanding the interface between the perceptions fat women have of themselves and the expectations and judgments society places on them. Regardless of how "healthy" these women or fat people in general are, my goal as a sociologist and feminist is to analyze (and expose) inequity and oppression within society.

Second, the biomedical research regarding the harms and health consequences of "obesity" is not as clear-cut as the media, politicians, and some physicians obstinately claim. Most of the research that is cited as "evidence" that fat causes ill health is *correlational* in nature and has not appropriately controlled for numerous other predictors of health problems, often because there are too many extraneous variables that are impossible to measure (see also Campos 2004; Oliver 2006). People whose body size falls at the extreme ends of the weight spectrum—both extremely thin and fat—are likely to suffer from health problems, but that does not mean that all fat people are unhealthy or that all thin or "normal"-sized people are healthy. So while I argue that the way "obesity" is framed in contemporary society is sensationalized and overblown, I do not claim that there are no health consequences for those at the larger end of the weight spectrum.

Part of the concern I have with the sensationalistic framing of "obesity" is that news sources frequently tout that "obesity" is quickly becoming the number one threat facing US citizens and that the growing number of fat Americans is causing a national crisis (Boero 2012; Saguy 2013). It is fascinating that these news sources rely on aggregate measures of "obesity," yet the solution is almost always framed as an individual problem (Oliver 2006). Of course, this is not unique to "obesity." Casper and Moore (2009), writing about infant mortality rates, eloquently discussed this irony: "We use aggregate data to measure and create problems through demographic truths, then fail to pursue *truly* aggregate (i.e., structural) solutions" (p. 72, emphasis in original). In other words, *if* "obesity" is a growing social problem, then the solutions should target structural issues that have led to this "social problem" rather than targeting people's individual bodies and practices, rendering fat people hypervisible "containers of blame" (Casper and Moore 2009). This perpetuates the mistreatment and discrimination of those who are fat, especially women and people of color. An increasing body of research clearly shows that fat shaming not only is ineffective as a method to "encourage" weight loss but has lasting and harmful physiological, psychological, and sociological consequences (Puhl and Heuer 2010; Schvey, Puhl, and Brownell 2014; Sutin and Terracciano 2013). The burgeoning field of Fat Studies has significantly elevated and expanded this conversation by increasing attention and scholarly study of the effects of fatphobia and stigmatization.

The Field of Fat Studies and the Present Study

I began conceptualizing this project in 2008, and since that time, the academic discipline of Fat Studies has begun to flourish.[4] Esther

Rothblum and Sandra Solovay published *The Fat Studies Reader* (2009) first. It was followed by *Fat Studies: An Interdisciplinary Journal of Body Weight and Society*. Moreover, sections and/or panels devoted to Fat Studies at academic conferences have grown or recently emerged. For instance, all the following associations have had sections devoted to Fat Studies in the last decade: Popular Culture Association (PCA), American Sociological Association (ASA), and the National Women's Studies Association (NWSA).[5] In 2007, when the call for papers was issued for the *Fat Studies Reader*, most people in mainstream sociology and feminism did not know what Fat Studies was, nor was it widely respected as an academic discipline (see the appendix for further discussion). The landscape is changing. In fact, as I have been writing this book, at least five academic books have been published in the field,[6] which speaks to the importance of the topic and the growing understanding that an increasing proportion of the population is being subjugated and Othered. In addition, these books have revealed that my findings are neither anomalous nor unique to the women I interviewed.

The Spectrum of Visibility and Hyper(in)visibility

These interviews revealed that having a fat body presents an *apparent* paradox because it is highly visible and publicly dissected and it is simultaneously marginalized and erased: It is hyper(in)visible. Contemporary Western societies relegate women who are fat to a hyper(in)visible space, a phenomenon that occurs explicitly within institutions and implicitly in our interpersonal worlds. The spectrum from hypervisible to hyperinvisible remains intense and deeply ingrained in our ceremonial social life. Therefore the prefix *hyper* is necessary to achieve the focus—the ocular ethic—necessary to analyze marginalized bodies, groups, or ways of life, because even though we all experience (in)visibility at times, one's situation becomes "hyper" when (in)visibility becomes socially oppressive.

Given how frequently fat women are mistreated in public, many were sensitive to even the most subtle stares or looks of disgust (cf. Tischner 2013). These experiences led to feelings of being persistently under the microscope, which in turn perpetuates their own self-discipline and surveillance (Foucault 1977). Moreover, the intense fatphobia that exists within the culture perpetuates the internalization of self-hatred and loathing that can lead to numerous physical and psychological problems. The majority of the women I interviewed have spent thousands of dollars and a tremendous amount of time trying to lose weight. They have avoided preventative care visits with physicians, have shunned engaging in social activities because of their size, and have endured mistreatment from strangers and loved ones alike. They have suffered hyper(in)visibility.

As I discussed in Chapter 1, visibility is linked to acknowledgement and recognition (Brighenti 2007). To be seen by another person is an indication that we exist. In addition, one of the ways we come to know who we are occurs as we examine and acknowledge how others see us through the societally constructed prism that identifies the "normal." We learn where we "stand" in the social hierarchy based on the way others locate us and view us in social and societal terms (Stone 1962, 87–88). Visibility is also tied to scrutiny or close inspection. If one has a bodily feature that makes him or her "stand out," then he or she is often the subject of disapproving stares.

Invisibility works similarly—it can be positive or negative. Privileged bodies are invisible in that they can easily move through the world without scrutiny or close inspection. As I wrote in Chapter 1, "Privileged bodies are visible when the situation suits them." If one has a "visually unobtrusive body" (Garland-Thomson 2004), he or she can move through situations with ease, but if one has a "visually obtrusive body," he or she will become visible at inopportune times but remain invisible when it is most important to be seen, such as when needing assistance. There is a dialectical relationship between visibility and invisibility (Star and Strauss 1999). However, I argue that the spectrum of visibility must include the two extremes of hypervisibility and hyperinvisibility to account for the *seemingly* paradoxical social position of marginalized bodies and persons. Marginalized bodies are not just acknowledged and seen; they are made into a spectacle. They are not simply invisible; they are frequently erased or dismissed from consideration.

The structural manifestation of hyper(in)visibility is present in the messages projected by the media, the medical establishment, and popular culture, while at the individual level women who are fat suffer further effects of hyper(in)visibility through social interactions infused with labeling, prejudice, and sizeism. In this way, fat women are both relegated to the social position of Other and sometimes relegated by themselves to this marginalized social position by "doing fat" (i.e., embodying fat stereotypes in social situations). I contend that hyper(in)visibility is a mode of Othering that subjugates fat women's—and other marginalized persons'—lived experiences and reinforces mistreatment and discrimination. Throughout this book, I have sought to make transparent the social oppression of women of size and to thematize the paradox of hyper(in)visibility.

I argue that the concept of hyper(in)visibility can be applied broadly to a variety of marginalized groups and bodies. For instance, those who are diagnosed as mentally ill are often hyper(in)visible. Structurally and experientially, those with mental-health problems such as schizophrenia or bipolar disorder are, for the most part, radically ignored and dismissed. Their needs are not acknowledged by the state, which often leads to homelessness, suicide, and sometimes incarceration. However, if someone who has been labeled mentally ill commits a violent crime, as we have seen in a number of the recent school shootings, the issues of mental health and mental illness become magnified and hypervisible, but only momentarily, and then the focus is removed and the issues of mental illness become hyperinvisible once again.

Other marginalized groups also suffer from the phenomenon of hyper(in)visibility. People who identify as lesbian, gay, bisexual, transgender, or queer experience hyper(in)visibility, as do rape and sexual assault victims, returning wounded soldiers, undocumented immigrants, those with disabilities or physical differences, and those who engage in extreme body modification. I contend that this concept has extensive applicability to marginalized bodies and groups and provides a framework to analyze both the structural aspects of oppression and denigration and the experiential aspects associated with the internalization of a marginalized status.

The stories and experiences that I have shared in this book are not necessarily generalizable to all women of size in North America, because (1) the women I interviewed self-selected to participate in this project, and (2) the sample was not as diverse as I hoped it would be (the majority of the women I interviewed identified as white and heterosexual). However, there are several factors that add validity and reliability to these data. First, the experiences recounted by the women I interviewed mirrored those I read in memoirs, autobiographies, listservs and blog posts, and other nonfiction works that focus on the lives or experiences of fat persons in contemporary society. Second, the sample was large enough that I was able to reach a point of theoretical saturation (Glaser and Strauss 1967), meaning that the data generated no new findings.

Nearly every woman that I spoke with told me that she responded to my call for participants because she was hoping that her story could help other women. Hopefully, this book will do that. But more research needs to be done. It is incredibly important for future researchers to continue to study the lives and experiences of those labeled fat. Future research should aim to select a more diverse sample in terms of race/ethnicity and sexual identity. In addition, one line worth pursuing is to investigate how men who are fat perceive their treatment in society, especially as the "war on obesity" escalates.

Shifting the Focus

I argue that, as a society, we need to move away from the obsession with thinness and appearance. One way this can be done is through education. First and foremost, educators could focus on media literacy. Children and adolescents should be taught how to read and decipher media messages, especially since most bodily images portrayed in advertisements have been edited and sculpted using computer software. Moreover, nutrition and health should be taught in a way that does not perpetuate harmful stereotypes for those who are at the larger end of the weight spectrum. Instead of demonizing large bodies, attention should be paid to eating whole, nutritionally dense foods and engaging in moderate activity (i.e., Health at Every Size®).

In a content analysis of high school textbooks, Jennings (2014) found that people of size were not only severely underrepresented but also stereotypically and negatively portrayed. She found that fatness was framed as incompatible with health and that some of the advice about weight management was contradictory and bordered on promoting disordered eating behaviors. Education should focus on healthful behaviors such as eating whole foods, getting moderate physical activity, and sleeping for seven to eight hours per night, rather than emphasizing body weight or body size.

Yet as the fear of fat grows, some schools have begun to send home report cards regarding the student's body mass index (BMI). The emphasis on body weight or having a specific body size can lead to weight cycling and potentially disordered eating. Research indicates that fat shaming, fatphobia, and the tremendous attention paid to the "obesity epidemic" fuels unhealthy dieting, increases rates of eating disorders, and can lead to negative health consequences (Darby et al. 2009, 2007).

Media representations of women of all sizes and shapes would also help promote diversity and more accurately represent contemporary women. Marian Wright Edelman, founder and president of the Children's Defense Fund, once said, "We can't be what we can't see." If young girls only see one female form depicted in the media—young, light skinned, thin, toned, large busted, and long legged—they might believe that that form is the only attractive and socially acceptable female form. Unfortunately, that representation of women misrepresents what the majority of the women in North America look like.

I closed the previous chapter with a discussion about a segment on the popular NPR show *Tell Me More* where the show's now deceased producer Teshima Walker Izrael asked for more complex roles for large women in film and television. There have only been a handful of women of size represented positively in the media in the last decade or so. For example, Melissa McCarthy, a woman of size, stars in the television show *Mike & Molly* and has been in popular films such as *Bridesmaids*, *The Heat*, and *Identity Thief*, to name a few. There have been a few women of size represented on popular television shows in a manner that does not play into simple stereotypes, but there have not been enough. Mostly, women who do not meet the extraordinarily narrow strictures of conventional beauty find themselves underrepresented in popular culture or typecast into the jovial, nonsexual fat woman or the overly emotional, desperate fat woman.

Finally, laws that prohibit weight discrimination should be adopted in more locales. Currently, laws exist in the following US locations: Madison (Wisconsin), Santa Cruz, San Francisco (both California), Urbana (Illinois), Washington, DC, and the state of Michigan. These laws function like other laws that prohibit discrimination based on race/ethnicity, sex/gender, sexuality, religion, and age (Schallenkamp, DeBeaumont, and Houy 2012). Numerous studies have found that those who are categorized as "obese" or "overweight" are paid less than their thinner counterparts (Averett and Korenman 1996; Baum and Ford 2004)—this effect has been found to be more profound for white women than women of color and men (Cawley 2004; Mason 2012; Register and Williams 1990)—and are less likely to be hired and promoted (Sartore and Cunningham 2007). Moreover, other research has found that women labeled "obese" tend to have lower academic achievement (Crosnoe 2007) and are less likely to marry higher-earning men, perpetuating the cycle of lower earnings (McEvoy 1992).

Research indicates that a key component to health and well-being is financial security (Ernsberger 2009). We often hear reports that poverty is fattening because those who are impoverished may have less access to healthful, nutritious foods and lack the time and resources to exercise due to long work hours with little compensation and benefits. Research shows that as a result they are exposed to higher levels of stress (which can raise cortisol levels and lead to weight gain; Schvey, Puhl, and Brownell 2014). However, there is some evidence to indicate that being fat leads to poverty, rather than the converse (Ernsberger 2009; Sorensen 1995). This is likely the result of discrimination and stigma, which can lead to unemployment and lower wages. If laws were in place across the United States to protect people of all body sizes, it is possible that some of this would correct itself, and theoretically, it would improve the health and well-being of those affected most—those labeled "obese."

In sum, throughout the book, I have employed Casper and Moore's (2009) ocular ethic to magnify fat bodies so that the social oppression of women who are fat becomes transparent and the phenomenon of hyper(in)visibility is no longer hidden. My hope is that by bringing this predicament to light through the voices of those who are oppressed, we as a society can begin to move away from harmful stereotypes and see people who are fat as human beings who deserve to be treated with dignity and respect—not deviant bodies.

Appendix
Notes on Methodology

As I noted in Chapter 1, this book began from my interest in "hogging." Recall that hogging is a practice where groups of men seek women they deem fat for sport or sexual gratification (Gailey and Prohaska 2006). Prior to that research, I was not familiar with Fat Studies or the size acceptance movement. It was through the hogging research that I began to understand how little research there was about women of size—especially their sexual experiences. The more I read about the mistreatment of people of size and the invisibility of fat women sexually, the more determined I became to design a project to address this lacuna.

I chose qualitative methods because this topic was relatively unexplored. Qualitative methods are typically used when little is known about a group or phenomenon. The goal of qualitative methods is to seek in-depth and intimate information from smaller groups of people rather than utilizing a large-scale study that seeks some form of verification. Qualitative researchers seek "thick description" (Geertz 1973) as opposed to answers to prearranged closed-ended questions. I focused on the specific method of in-depth interviews because I wanted to listen to women's stories but be able to interject and probe for follow-up or more detail if they glossed over an issue. Moreover, I utilized participant observation on listservs, social networking groups, and other online forums so that I could immerse myself in the population—as best as possible—to get a sense of the issues affecting persons of size and subsequent discourse surrounding these issues.

This book is based on two sets of in-depth interviews with 74 North American women and the observation of multiple online groups and listservs. The inclusion criteria for both sets of interviews were women over 18 with a body mass index (BMI) greater than or equal to 30 ("obese"). I chose to use BMI as a criterion because I did not want to make subjective decisions about who was "fat enough" to participate. The women's ages ranged from 19 to 62, and 5 identified as Latina, 1 as mixed ethnicity Latina, 1 as Native American, 6 as African American, 1 as Gambian West African, and 60 as Caucasian, 2 of whom Canadian. Their weights ranged from 170 pounds to 550 pounds, with an average BMI of 45.9. This sample of women was fairly well educated, with only 3 women reporting their highest education level as high school or general equivalency; 18 women had completed some college, 2 had associates' degrees, 29 had bachelor's degrees, 13 had master's degrees, 3 had juris doctorates and were practicing lawyers, and 6 had doctor of philosophy degrees (PhDs). In terms of relationship status, 34 women reported that they were single, 2 were engaged, 5 indicted that they were partnered and cohabitating, 17 were married, 15 were divorced, and 1 was a widow.

In 2009, I recruited women of size from a variety of sources that were all related to size acceptance. I chose that selection method because, at the time, I was not sure how else to go about recruiting women who were likely to have experienced weight-based discrimination or that most would consider fat. I used multiple listservs, websites, blogs, and the National Association to Advance Fat Acceptance (NAAFA) to spread the word about the project. Originally I was hoping to talk with women about their dating and sexual histories and involvement, if any, in the size acceptance movement, but it became much more than that.

I should also mention that initially I had some difficulty getting women to agree to talk with me because of my university affiliation. Many of the folks were concerned that I represented the religious right and that I would use the information they shared "as proof that fat women are deviant." For the majority of the those who did agree to participate, I spent quite a bit of time prior to the interview and their signing the consent document communicating with them about who I am, why I was studying this, what I was going to do with the research, and why I cared (especially as a woman who by most standards would not be considered fat), and I often provided a description of my university's policy on academic freedom.

In 2009 I recruited 36 women of size from size acceptance listservs, social networking groups, and/or size acceptance blogs. Of these women, 23 indicated that they "aren't that involved" in the size acceptance movement but do subscribe to blogs, social networking sites, and/or listservs; 8 were slightly more involved in the movement as writers, artists, researchers, or academics, and 5 identified as fat activists.

Nearly all the interviews took place over the phone, and each woman gave me permission to record the interview. The interviews lasted between 45 minutes and two and a half hours. It became clear to me as I started interviewing these women that there was so much more to discuss than simply their dating and sexual histories. In fact, when I asked women about their body image, they frequently spent a significant amount of time discussing the influence of their parents, siblings, grandparents, teachers, and peers.

I published only one paper from that set of interviews, and I think that is because I had a hard time removing myself from their stories and their pain. I was naïve, and I did not expect their lives to impact me the way they did. Some of the phone calls and stories still echo in my mind, particularly those early conversations where it was a challenge for me to "see" their experiences as data.

Another issue I faced was that as I submitted the initial paper to journals for publication, reviewers were suspicious about who the women were and if they were "fat enough" (because I did not include the women's weight range). One reviewer actually said, "Most women think they are fat, even when they aren't. Considering the high degree of confidence exuded by the women in this study I would need to know exactly how much these women weigh to even consider if the author's findings are credible." Another reviewer said, "I think the most important finding from this paper is that there are actually people out there who like to have sex with fat women" (anonymous referee comments for a scholarly journal). Both of these reviewers indicated that fat is ugly, not sexy, and that it was difficult to imagine that fat women could be confident and feel good about their bodies. I eventually published the paper at the newly founded journal *Fat Studies*, and it appeared in the inaugural issue (Gailey 2012). Such experiences made it clear to me that publishing this material was going to be difficult, but it also made me more determined to find an outlet to showcase these women's voices and stories.

In 2012, I expanded my recruiting techniques because I wanted to find women who likely knew nothing about size acceptance as a point of comparison. I posted a call for participants on Craigslist, various Yahoo! groups, and on my personal Facebook page and asked friends to share the post. I also asked participants to spread the word about the study to their friends and family, which resulted in a couple of people contacting me, but not as many as I had hoped. Many of the women said they knew women who would likely participate, but they did not want to suggest it to their friend because that would mean that they were "calling their friend fat." I left it up to each individual woman to contact her friend, if she so wished, and made it clear that the friend should contact me if interested. Several did, but most were not comfortable doing so.

I also contacted several bariatric surgery support groups at local hospitals. One of the group coordinators invited me to give a lecture to the group after she read the *Fat Studies* article (Gailey 2012). Following my presentation, I told the group that I was recruiting women of size for in-depth interviews because I was studying the treatment of fat women in society. I left my contact information for them if they were interested. I was able to recruit two women from that event. In the end, I interviewed an additional 38 women in 2012. Only 3 of the 38 women identified with the size acceptance ideology, but all expressed histories of internalized fat oppression, similar to the majority of the women in the first set of interviews.

The second set of interviews also consisted of telephone and in-person interviews. Approximately two-thirds of the interviews were conducted over the phone and the remaining one-third were done face to face, usually in my home or at my office. These interviews tended to last a little longer than the first 36, with a range of an hour and fifteen minutes to four and a half hours. I offered to meet participants in any location, but almost all chose my house, and several wanted to come to my office. Only one woman invited me to her house.

Across both sets of interviews, when participants saw my recruitment letter or were notified by a friend about the study, they made the initial contact via email. I responded to each email with more information about the study and attached two consent documents: (1) agreement to participate in the interview and (2) agreement to allow me record the interview. In addition to sending the form electronically, I also offered to mail participants the documents (two copies of each) as well as a self-addressed postage-paid envelope. Several women took me up on that offer, but most did not. Most of the women either signed the forms and sent them back electronically or mailed them to my work address.

At the beginning of each interview, I asked them if they had any concerns or questions about the project. I also asked their permission to turn on the recorder, and at the end of the interview I notified them that I was turning off the recorder. Some of the women continued to talk with me after I stopped recording, but usually not for very long, and it typically consisted of things like them asking me what I was going to do with the findings and if they could read it when I was through.

I began each interview by asking the women demographic-type questions such as their race/ethnicity, age, marital status, and if they went to college. The question about education typically turned into a discussion about how their weight impacted them in school (both grade school and college). Most of the women who agreed to talk with me wanted to tell someone their story. They wanted people to know what has been hard for them, what has worked, and sometimes where they hope to be in the future. But it was really important to almost all of them that this project be honest so that it would "help other fat women."

There were not discernable differences between the in-person and phone interviews. The in-person interviews lasted just as long as the phone interviews, the amount of information the participants revealed was similar, and the interactions were not remarkably different. I thought initially that it might be easier for the women to participate in a phone interview, especially because I am not a large woman, but that did not seem to matter. The women I interviewed face to face were forthright and open, which is evident by the personal nature of the information they revealed to me.

One concern I had about the phone interviews was that it might seem too impersonal or that the participant would become distracted by family members, pets, television, and so forth. This was surprisingly not the case. There were some minor interruptions, such as someone calling in on the other line, in one case a small child in the background, and plenty of barking dogs and meowing cats, but nothing that took the attention away from the interview. In most cases, it gave us something to laugh about and provided a bit of a relief from the emotionally intense conversation.

I asked each woman if she wanted me to contact her when I had completed the project and nearly all said yes. Of those who expressed interest, I noted their email addresses and contacted them when I finished writing this book.

All interviews were in-depth and semistructured. I had questions prepared in advance to keep the interviews focused, but additional questions were asked as a result of the conversations. I wanted the women to feel at ease sharing, and most were forthright and quite talkative. The average interview, during both data collection points, was 2 hours and 25 minutes.

In addition to the two sets of interviews, I also read numerous memoirs, autobiographies, and other nonfiction books about the lives of people of size. I subscribe to several "people of size" listservs and am connected to Fat Studies and size acceptance groups on Facebook. In other words, I have spent the last several years reading threaded discussions and posts, articles that members post or recommend, and books written by members or those who many members highly admire. Immersing myself in the "fat-o-sphere" and size acceptance community has helped me gain a greater understanding of the needs, issues, and lives of the women I interviewed.

I used grounded theory for the data analysis. Grounded theory is a technique where the researcher codes the data as it is collected in order to utilize theoretical sampling, a process whereby the researcher seeks information on themes that arise from the subsequent participants. As patterns and themes emerged from the interviews, additional questions were asked in the subsequent interviews, to further tease out the distinctions until a theoretical model developed and a point of saturation was achieved, meaning the data yielded no new findings (Glaser and Strauss 1967).

Throughout the course of both sets of interviews and observations that took place over several years, various themes and patterns materialized. As I examined the interview transcripts, blogs, bulletins, posts, comments, and forums, I coded these data into manageable content categories such as fat shame, bodily acceptance, disordered eating, health problems, diets, family relationships, fear, hatred, and so forth. Therefore, whenever any of the concepts were mentioned, I coded the text accordingly. As the analysis and coding progressed, it became clear that some of the concepts were used together and some occurred much more frequently than others. I had to tease out the subtle distinctions to determine which themes were the most inclusive.

All the women indicated that they had experienced some form of mistreatment or discrimination. They also all discussed their stories on what I call a spectrum of visibility. For instance, they mentioned feeling dismissed or invisible, or they talked about walking down the street and often simultaneously experiencing the sensation of being "on stage"—a direct result of the weight of people's stares. I argue that the phenomenon of hyper(in)visibility is the bridge that connects and traverses the diverse themes that emerged throughout my discussions with participants about their experiences as fat women.

Throughout the book, I situate the emerging themes of these women's experiences as fat women in a cultural and political context, but I do not claim scientific objectivity. I follow both poststructuralist and interactionist research epistemologies that have discredited such claims (Denzin 1989; Haraway 2000). I studied the discourse these women used to understand their position in society, gain acceptance, and cope in a fatphobic culture, but I also tried to understand their lives from the critical perspectives of fat studies, feminism, symbolic interactionism, and poststructuralism. These theoretical perspectives have shaped my interests and focus. They initially led me to question the hyperbolic messages surrounding fat and the way fat women are subsequently treated, and they later guided my exploration of the struggles over acceptance, dieting, mistreatment, oppression, health, medicine, pleasure, sexuality, and body politics that play out in these women's lives.

Equalizing the Interview

The feminist tradition of equalizing the interviews calls on researchers to make the interview setting less asymmetrical, wherein the interviewer has all the power and the interviewee has little or none. One of the reasons many feminist academics, myself included, are concerned about this is because often the groups that academics study have less social capital and privilege than the researcher. This is referred to as "studying down." Because feminism as an ideology seeks equality among men and women, racial and ethnic groups, varying social class positions, and so forth, it is disconcerting to engage in research with people who tend to have less social privilege and ask them to give everything while the researcher reveals nothing (Oakley 1981; Sinding and Aronson 2003).

Agreeing to an interview about one's life and specifically one's body is intimate, and I was concerned that the women I spoke with would feel like the interaction was one-sided. I did not want them to feel exploited. In an attempt to equalize the interview, I answered any and all questions participants had about my personal life. The questions that were most commonly asked included things like if I had ever been fat, whether I have body image issues, how much I currently weigh, have I ever been made fun for my weight, do I have fat people in my family or who I care deeply for, what will I do with their information, why am I interested in this topic, and so forth.

To give the reader some perspective of how I answered their questions, I told the women that I have never been fat, but I felt like I was for most of my life. Physically, I developed very quickly as a child and before my most of my peers. In fact, I developed so quickly that by seventh grade I had reached my adult size. Actually, I weighed more in seventh grade than I do in my late thirties. Because I developed so quickly, I was incredibly self-conscious about my body. I felt huge and I thought other kids thought I was, too. However, in hindsight I realize that judgment was likely false.

I strove to make the interview experience equal by treating respondents as equals. I offered support throughout the interviews and shared information that I thought might be helpful. For instance, several women noted that they could not find active wear in their size, and I told them the names of stores that were frequently mentioned on blogs or listservs. Other women wanted to know if others I had spoken with had similar experiences or if they were alone, and I assured them that there were others who had had similar experiences and sometimes even shared small bits of other women's stories (of course without mentioning names or revealing information).

It was not uncommon for interviewees to cry at some point during the interview. When this happened, I always asked them if they wanted to continue and if they were OK, and in one instance, I changed the subject so that the participant could talk about a happier time in her life. She later returned to the initial conversation when she was ready.

It was not uncommon for me to cry following an interview that was particularly difficult. In fact, almost all the interviews affected me quite dramatically. For instance, following some interviews, I was completely exhausted and depleted of energy, whereas following others I felt invigorated and motivated. I was able to establish good rapport with all the women, and I think that they ultimately trusted me with their story. In fact, numerous women shared stories with me that they said they have never shared with anyone else. Many of the women also sent me follow-up emails thanking me, filling in information they had forgotten, or asking me how the project was progressing. Most of the women thanked me at the end of the interview and said that the experience was cathartic.

Throughout the book, I strove to accurately and adequately represent the voices of the women who agreed to speak with me and who I have observed via threaded discussions, social networking, and through reading various nonfiction books about the lives of people of size. I hope that my interpretation and analysis is useful academically to my colleagues and, more important, personally for the participants and other women of size.

Notes

Chapter 1

1. All participants' names throughout the book are pseudonyms to ensure confidentiality.
2. I use the term *fat* here as an adjective in the spirit of size acceptance and not as a derogatory term.
3. *The Biggest Loser*, NBC Official Site. http://www.biggestloser.com. Accessed on October 5, 2012.
4. "Biggest Loser: Contestants Admit Dangerous Practices, Can't Speak Out." *Huffington Post*, November 25, 2009. http://www.huffingtonpost.com/2009/11/25/biggest-loser contestants_n_370538.html. Accessed April 10, 2010.
5. "The Weight of the Nation: Films." HBO. http://theweightofthenation.hbo.com/films. Accessed on October 5, 2012.
6. In June 2013, the American Medical Association voted to officially label "obesity" a disease.
7. NAAFA website. http://www.naafa.org. Accessed October 5, 2012.

Chapter 2

1. Hannele Harjunen and Katariina Kyrölä have also written about fat as a temporary status or something separate from the body. For instance, Kyrölä (2014) has discussed fat as a "phantom limb," and Harjunen (2009) has discussed fat as a "liminal" state.
2. I discuss the idea of embracing or embodying one's fat in greater detail in Chapter 6.
3. Some of the women discussed the idea of passing as thin when they talked about trying to wear things that covered their fat, such as baggy shirts. One woman said, "I used to wear clothes that were too big to try to hide my belly, as if I could pass as thin." But the concept was also discussed by a few women who had at one point in their lives lost a tremendous amount of weight. They had a difficult time embodying their thinness because they still saw themselves as fat. They said they felt like they were trying to "pass" as thin.
4. Cahnman (1968) published an article in *Sociological Quarterly* about the stigma of obesity. There were few others writing at the time about

the relationship, but it does show that being fat has carried a tremendous social burden for at least the last fifty years.
5. I describe the various weight-loss surgery procedures, including lap band, in more detail in Chapter 3.
6. Polycystic ovary syndrome (PCOS) is a hormonal disorder that affects women of reproductive age. According to Mayo Clinic, women who have PCOS typically have enlarged ovaries that contain numerous cysts. The symptoms of PCOS include excess hair growth, acne, infrequent or irregular periods, and unexplained weight gain.
7. The Strong4Life and the Children's Healthcare of America campaign were launched in Georgia to "eradicate childhood obesity" (see also Gray 2012 and Teegardin 2012).
8. Unfortunately there is not extensive research regarding intimate partner violence and women of size, but there are several pieces devoted to the subject—for instance, see Koppelman 2003 and Royce 2009. I also discuss some forms of abuse by intimate partners in Chapter 5.
9. I discuss Liz's and other women's perspectives about fat, health, and fitness in Chapter 4.

Chapter 3

1. I discuss PCOS and hypothyroidism in Chapter 4.
2. There are reasons to be concerned about adolescents taking amphetamines: (1) they might become addicted, and (2) some research indicates that amphetamine use in adolescence can alter the brain's functioning in adulthood, even when the person no longer is taking the drug. "Adolescent Amphetamine Use Linked to Permanent Changes in Brain Function and Behavior." McGill University Health Centre, November 3, 2011. http://muhc.ca/newsroom/news/adolescent-amphetamine-use-linked-permanent-changes-brain-function-and-behaviour. Accessed on April 29, 2012.
3. According to Mayo Clinic, the risks and complications associated with lap band procedures include band slippage, which requires another surgery, gall stones, stomach perforation, dehydration, malnutrition, no weight loss, and so on, not to mention the physical risk inherent in having a surgical procedure.
4. "Nutrition and Weight Management." Boston Medical Center website. http://www.bmc.org/nutritionweight/services/weightmanagement.htm. Accessed on May 3, 2012.
5. "100 Million Dieters, $20 Billion: The Weight-Loss Industry by the Numbers." ABC News, May 8, 2012. http://abcnews.go.com/Health/100-million-dieters-20-billion-weight-loss-industry/story?id=16297197. Accessed on May 8, 2012.

6. "U.S. Weight Loss Market Forecast to Hit $66 Billion in 2013." PRWeb, December 31, 2012. http://www.prweb.com/releases/2012/12/prweb10278281.htm. Accessed on January 29, 2013.
7. This does not account for those who are unable to participate due to childcare demands or because the cost is too high.
8. American Psychological Association website. http://www.apa.org. Accessed on January 15, 2013.
9. Mayo Clinic website. http://www.MayoClinic.org. Accessed on January 14, 2013.
10. Healthful eating most frequently referred to eliminating processed and fast foods and sticking to a diet that consisted of whole foods. I discuss health and healthy eating in more detail in Chapter 4.
11. In the myth of Sisyphus, the gods punish Sisyphus by sentencing him to an eternity of pushing a large rock up a mountain; upon reaching the top, the rock would roll back to the bottom and Sisyphus would have to start over (Camus 1955).

CHAPTER 4

1. "International Classification of Diseases (ICD)." World Health Organization. http://www.who.int/classifications/icd/en. Accessed on November 15, 2013.
2. "The Rudd Center Health Digest, June 2013." Yale Rudd Center for Food Policy and Obesity. http://www.yaleruddcenter.org/newsletter/issue.aspx?id=58. Accessed on October 2, 2013.
3. For the full story, see "Type Miscast: An Elmhurst Doctor's Type 2 Diabetes Misdiagnosis Results in the Death of a Six-Year-Old Girl." *The Village Voice*, October 2, 2013. http://www.villagevoice.com/2013-10-02/news/type-2-diabetes-misdiagnosis-kills-six-year-old-girl-dr-arlene-mercado-claudialee-gomez-nicanor. Accessed on October 3, 2013.
4. See Chapter 3 for a discussion about the risks associated with weight-loss medication and weight-loss surgery.
5. "What to Say at the Doctor's Office." Ragen Chastain's blog, *Dances with Fat*, April 1, 2013. http://danceswithfat.wordpress.com/2013/04/01/what-to-say-at-the-doctors-office. Accessed on October 20, 2013.
6. For a more detailed explanation of the condition, see Lymphedema Therapy website. http://www.lymphedema-therapy.com/Lipedema.htm. Accessed on October 21, 2013.
7. Catherine Seo. "Lipoedema: You Mean It's Not My Fault?" http://youtu.be/ncvw-SwWk5Q. Accessed on November 10, 2013.

8. "Death by Stigma: Why We Must Stop Weight Stigma." Binge Eating Disorder Association. http://bedaonline.com/death-by-stigma-why-we-must-stop-weight-stigma. Accessed on November 3, 2013.
9. "Your Fat Is (Allegedly) Killing You!!!: Weight Stigma and the Dangerous Nocebo Effect." Golda Poretsky's blog. http://www.bodylovewellness.com/2013/09/23/your-fat-is-allegedly-killing-you-weight-stigma-and-the-dangerous-nocebo-effect. Accessed on November 22, 2013.

Chapter 5

1. There are two books that have been published about sex and persons of size that are not scholarly. One is Hanne Blank's (2000) *Big Big Love: A Sex and Relationships Guide for People of Size (and Those Who Love Them)*, and the other is Rebecca Jane Weinstein's (2012) *Fat Sex: The Naked Truth*.
2. See Chapter 4 for a discussion about health and weight and a discussion about researchers who perpetuate the idea that one's weight is an individual choice.
3. "The Weight of the Nation: Films." HBO. http://theweightofthenation.hbo.com. Accessed January 12, 2014.
4. A number of the women I interviewed for this project were at one time thin because they lost enough weight that they no longer met the medical criteria for "overweight" or "obesity." They discussed feeling like they were fake or not in their real body. A few also reported that they did not like the attention that their body warranted when they were thinner.

Chapter 6

1. For discussions about the conflation of thinness and beauty, see Bordo (1993), Chernin (1994), and Wolf ([1991] 2002).
2. See Cooper 1998, 2012; Farrell 2009; and Saguy 2013 for excellent summaries and discussions about the movement.
3. Some argue that NAAFA, in particular, prizes fat bodies over thin bodies and creates a new form of sizeism. Some of the women I interviewed even said they did not feel comfortable at NAAFA functions because they were at the smaller end of the fat spectrum and they felt like outsiders or ignored by those who were at the larger end of the weight spectrum. Just like any social movement, it is not monolithic, and different views and priorities are stressed depending on whom or which group one speaks with (I discuss this in some detail toward the end of this chapter). Moreover, NAAFA is not the only formal size acceptance organization. Two others are the Canadian Association for

Size Acceptance (CASA) and the International Size Acceptance Association (ISAA).
4. NAAFA website. http://www.naafaonline.com/dev2/about/NEWSLETTERS.html. Accessed December 13, 2013.
5. This discussion reminds me of the ongoing debate in the women's movement about whether the word *feminist* should be replaced with the word *humanist* because feminism carries so many negative connotations in mainstream culture.
6. "NAAFA Constitution." http://www.naafaonline.com/dev2/about/byLaws/Constitution-VER09.pdf. Accessed December 21, 2013.
7. Angela Son. "Fat Activist Brenda Oelbaum." *The Ground Magazine*, August 28, 2013. http://www.thegroundmag.com/fat-activist-brenda-oelbaum. Accessed December 13, 2013.
8. Sally E. Smith. "Fat Enough to Belong." *Dimensions Magazine*. http://www.dimensionsmagazine.com/dimtext/ses/ses74.html. Accessed May 23, 2014.
9. For a discussion of this term, see the blog post on *Shapely Prose* written by Sweet Machine, September 5, 2007: http://kateharding.net/2008/10/30/from-the-archives-fat-acceptance-and-the-acceptance-of-fat. Accessed May 23, 2014.
10. Thank you to Michaela Nowell for helping me better understand the nuance associated with weight tensions in the size acceptance movement.
11. Michel Martin. "Remembering Tell Me More's Teshima Walker Izrael." National Public Radio, August 26, 2013. http://www.npr.org/templates/story/story.php?storyId=215764268&utm_medium=Email&utm_source=share&utm_campaign. Accessed March 28, 2014.

Chapter 7

1. It harms men, too. Men are increasingly objectified and held to higher standards regarding their appearance and physique, but it is different, and at the time I am writing this book, it still disproportionately affects women.
2. Robin Erb. "Student Takes on Prejudice against Overweight People." *USA Today*, December 29, 2013. http://www.usatoday.com/story/news/nation/2013/12/29/battle-body-hate-student-politics/4235001. Accessed on December 29, 2013.
3. "Normalizing Obesity." Ragen Chastain's blog, *Dances with Fat*, December 30, 2013. http://danceswithfat.wordpress.com/2013/12/30/normalizing-obesity. Accessed on January 15, 2014.
4. The field of Fat Studies began much earlier with several instrumental publications such as *Shadow on a Tightrope: Writings by Women on Fat*

Oppression edited by Lisa Schoenfielder and Barb Wieser in 1983 and *Such a Pretty Face: Being Fat in America* by Marcia Millman, published in 1980. See Charlotte Cooper's (2012) piece in the *Fat Studies Journal* for a complete history of fat activism.
5. This list is not meant to be exhaustive but instead represents conferences that I, as a sociologist, am familiar with and would have the opportunity to be involved in and present my work.
6. *Killer Fat* (2012; Natalie Boero), *Framing Fat* (2013; Samantha Kwan and Jennifer Graves), *Fat* (2013; Deborah Lupton), *What's Wrong with Fat* (2013; Abigail Saguy), and *Fat Lives* (2013; Irmgard Tischner).

References

Alexander, C. Normal, and Mary Glenn Wiley. 1981. "Situated Activity and Identity Formation." In *Social Psychology: Sociological Perspectives*, edited by M. Rosenberg and R. Turner, 269–89. New York: Basic.

American Psychiatric Association. 2013. *Diagnostic and Statistical Manual of Mental Disorders*, 5th edition. Washington, DC: American Psychiatric Association.

Amy, Nancy K., Annette E. Aalborg, Pat Lyons, and Laura Keranen. 2006. "Barriers to Routine Gynecological Cancer Screening for White and African-American Obese Women." *International Journal of Obesity*, 30: 147–55.

Andreyeva, Tatiana, Rebecca M. Puhl, and Kelly D. Brownell. 2008. "Changes in Perceived Weight Discrimination among Americans, 1995–1996 through 2004–2006." *Obesity*, 16 (5): 1129–34.

Armstrong, D. 1995. "The Rise of Surveillance Medicine." *Sociology of Health and Illness*, 17 (3): 393–404.

Averett, Susan, and Sanders Korenman. 1996. "The Economic Reality of the Beauty Myth." *Journal of Human Resources*, 31 (2): 304–30.

Bacon, Linda. 2010. *Health at Every Size: The Surprising Truth about Your Weight*, 2nd edition. Dallas: BenBella.

Bagley, C. R., D. N. Conklin, R. T. Isherwood, D. R. Pechiulis, and L. A. Watson. 1989. "Attitudes of Nurses toward Obesity and Obese Patients." *Perception Motor Skills*, 68: 954.

Baum, Charles, and William Ford. 2004. "The Wage Effects of Obesity: A Longitudinal Study." *Health Economics*, 13 (9): 885–99.

Beauboeuf-Lafontant, Tamara. 2003. "Strong and Large Black Women? Exploring Relationships between Deviant Womanhood and Weight." *Gender & Society*, 17 (1): 111–21.

Becker, M. 1986. "The Tyranny of Health Promotion." *Public Health Review*, 14: 15–25.

Berg, Frances M. 1999. "Health Risk Associated with Weight Loss and Obesity Treatment Programs." *Journal of Social Issues*, 55 (2): 277–97.

Bjorntorp, P., K. De Jounge, L. Sjorstorm, and N. Kleim. 1970. "The Effect of Physical Training on Insulin Production in Obesity." *Metabolism*, 19: 631–38.

Blank, Hanne. 2000. *Big Big Love: A Sourcebook on Sex for People of Size and Those Who Love Them*. Emeryville, CA: Greenery.
Blumberg, P., and L. P. Mellis. 1980. "Medical Students' Attitudes toward the Obese and Morbidly Obese." *International Journal of Eating Disorders*, 4: 169–75.
Boero, Natalie. 2012. *Killer Fat: Media, Medicine, and Morals in the American "Obesity Epidemic."* New Brunswick, NJ: Rutgers University Press.
Bordo, Susan. 1993. *Unbearable Weight: Feminism, Western Culture, and the Body*. Berkeley: University of California Press.
Bouchard, C., A. Tremblay, J. P. Després, A. Nadeau, P. J. Lupien, G. Thériault, J. Dussault, S. Moorjani, S. Pinault, and G. Fournier. 1990. "The Response to Long-Term Overfeeding in Identical Twins." *New England Journal of Medicine*, 322: 1477–82.
Braziel, Jana Evans. 2001. "Sex and Fat Chics: Deterritorializing the Fat Female Body." In *Bodies Out of Bounds*, edited by Jana Evans Braziel and Kathleen LeBesco, 231–54. Berkeley: University of California Press.
Brighenti, Andrea. 2007. "Visibility: A Category for the Social Sciences." *Current Sociology*, 55: 323–42.
Brittingham, Kim. 2011. *Read My Hips: How I Learned to Love My Body, Ditch Dieting, and Live Large*. New York: Three Rivers.
Burgard, Deb. 2009. "What Is 'Health at Every Size?'" In *The Fat Studies Reader*, edited by Esther Rothblum and Sandra Solovay, 42–53. New York: New York University Press.
Butler, Judith. 1993. *Bodies That Matter: On the Discursive Limits of "Sex."* New York: Routledge.
———. 1990. *Gender Trouble: Feminism and the Subversion of Identity*. New York: Routledge.
Cahnman, Werner J. 1968. "The Stigma of Obesity." *The Sociological Quarterly*, 9 (3): 283–99.
Campos, Paul. 2004. *The Obesity Myth: Why America's Obsession with Weight Is Hazardous to Your Health*. New York: Gotham.
Campos, Paul, Abigail Saguy, Paul Ernsberger, Eric Oliver, and Glenn Gaesser. 2006. "The Epidemiology of Overweight and Obesity: Public Health Crisis or Moral Panic?" *International Journal of Epidemiology*, 35 (1): 55–60.
Camus, Albert. 1955. *The Myth of Sisyphus*. New York: Alfred A. Knopf.
Cao, Sissi, Rahim Moineddin, Marcelo L. Urquia, Fahad Razak, and Joel G. Ray. 2014. "J-Shapedness: An Often Missed, Often Miscalculated Relation: The Example of Weight and Mortality." *Journal of Epidemiology and Community Health*, 68: 683–90. Accessed March 28, 2014: doi:10.1136/jech-2013-203439
Casper, Monica J., and Lisa Jean Moore. 2009. *Missing Bodies: The Politics of Visibility*. New York: New York University Press.
Cassuto, J., A. Feher, L. Lan, V. S. Patel, V. Kamath, D. C. Anthony, and Z. Bagi. 2013. "Obesity and Statins Are Both Independent Predictors of

Enhanced Coronary Arteriolar Dilation in Patients Undergoing Heart Surgery." *Journal of Cardiothoracic Surgery*, 8 (1): 117.
Cawley, J. 2004. "The Impact of Obesity on Wages." *Journal of Human Resources*, 39 (2): 451–74.
Cawley, J., and C. Meyerhoefer. 2012. "The Medical Care Costs of Obesity: An Instrumental Variables Approach." *Journal of Health Economics*, 31: 219–30.
Chernin, Kim. 1994. *The Obsession: Reflections on the Tyranny of Slenderness*. New York: Harper Perennial.
Cogan, Jeanine C. 1999. "Re-Evaluating the Weight-Centered Approach toward Health: The Need for a Paradigm Shift." In *Interpreting Weight: The Social Management of Fatness and Thinness*, edited by Jeffrey Sobal and Donna Maurer, 229–53. New York: Aldine De Gruyter.
Cogan, Jeanine C., and Paul Ernsberger. 1999. "Dieting, Weight, and Health: Reconceptualizing Research and Policy." *Journal of Social Issues*, 55 (2): 198–205.
Colberg, Sheri R., Ronald J. Sigal, Bo Fernhall, Judith G. Regensteiner, Bryan J. Blissmer, Richard R. Rubin, Lisa Chasan-Taber, Ann L. Albright, and Barry Braun. 2010. "Exercise and Type 2 Diabetes." *Diabetes Care*, 33: 147–67. Accessed November 16, 2013: doi: 10.2337/dc10-9990
Collins, Patricia Hill. 1990. *Black Feminist Thought: Knowledge, Consciousness, and the Politics of Empowerment*. New York: HarperCollins.
Connell, R. W. 1987. *Gender and Power*. Stanford, CA: Stanford University Press.
Conrad, Peter. 1992. "Medicalization and Social Control." *Annual Review of Sociology*, 18: 209–32.
———. 1987. "Wellness in the Workplace: Potentials and Pitfalls of Worksite Health Promotion." *Milbank Quarterly*, 65: 255–75.
Conrad, Peter, and Joseph W. Schneider. 1992. *Deviance and Medicalization: From Badness to Sickness*, 2nd edition. Philadelphia: Temple University Press.
Cooley, Charles Horton. 1902. *Human Nature and the Social Order*. New York: Scribner.
Cooper, Charlotte. 2012. "A Queer and Trans Fat Activist Timeline: Queering Fat Activist Nationality and Cultural Imperialism." *Fat Studies: An Interdisciplinary Journal of Body Weight and Society*, 1 (1): 61–74.
———. 2009. "The Story of the Chubsters." Paper presented at the Annual Conference of the National Popular Culture and American Culture Associations, April 11, New Orleans, LA.
———. 1998. *Fat and Proud: The Politics of Size*. London: Women's.
Courtot, Martha. 1983. "A Spoiled Identity." In *Shadow on a Tightrope: Writings by Women on Fat Oppression*, edited by Lisa Schoenfielder and Barb Wieser, 199–203. Iowa City, IA: Aunt Lute.

Crandall, C. S. 1994. "Prejudice against Fat People: Ideology and Self Interest." *Journal of Personality and Social Psychology*, 66 (5): 882–94.
Crawford, Robert. 1980. "Healthism and the Medicalization of Everyday Life." *International Journal of Health Services*, 10: 365–88.
Crosnoe, Robert. 2007. "Gender, Obesity, and Education." *Sociology of Education*, 80: 241–60.
Cross, W. E., Jr. 1991. *Shades of African American: Diversity in African-American Identity*. Philadelphia: Temple University Press.
Darby, Anita, Phillipa Hay, Jonathan Mond, Frances Quirk, Petra Buttner, and Lee Kennedy. 2009. "The Rising Prevalence of Comorbid Obesity and Eating Disorder Behaviors from 1995–2005." *International Journal of Eating Disorder*, 42: 104–8.
Darby, A., P. Hay, J. Mond, B. Rodgers, and C. Owen. 2007. "Disordered Eating Behaviors and Cognitions in Young Women with Obesity: Relationship with Psychological Status." *International Journal of Obesity*, 31: 876–82.
DeAngelis, Tory. 1997. "Body-Image Problems Affect All Groups." *Monitor on Psychology*, 28 (3): 45.
Denzin, Norman K. 1989. *Interpretive Biography*, vol. 17. Newbury Park, CA: Sage.
Dion, Karen K. 1972. "Physical Attractiveness and Evaluation of Children's Transgressions." *Journal of Personality and Social Psychology*, 24: 207–13.
Dion, Karen K., Ellen Berscheid, and Elaine Walster. 1972. "What Is Beautiful Is Good." *Journal of Personality and Social Psychology*, 24: 285–90.
Dolezal, Luna. 2010. "The (In)visible Body: Feminism, Phenomenology, and the Case of Cosmetic Surgery." *Hypatia*, 25: 357–75.
Ernsberger, Paul. 2012. "BMI, Body Build, Body Fatness, and Health Risks." *Fat Studies*, 1: 6–12.
———. 2009. "Does Social Class Explain the Connection between Weight and Health?" In *The Fat Studies Reader*, edited by Esther Rothblum and Sandra Solovay, 25–36. New York: New York University Press.
Ernsberger, Paul, and P. Haskew. 1987. "Health Implications of Obesity: An Alternative View." *Journal of Obesity and Weight Regulation*, 6: 58–137.
Farrell, Amy. 2011. *Fat Shame: Stigma and the Fat Body in American Culture*. New York: New York University Press.
Fee, Holly R., and Michael R. Nusbaumer. 2012. "Social Distance and the Formerly Obese: Does the Stigma of Obesity Linger?" *Sociological Inquiry*, 82: 1–22.
Fenske, Sarah. 2004. "Big Game Hunters. Men Who Chase Chubbies for Sport and Pleasure: They Call It Hogging." *Cleveland Scene Magazine*, 34: 15–18.
Field, A. E., S. B. Austin, C. B. Taylor, S. Malspeis, B. Rosner, H. R. Rockett, M. S. Gillman, and G. A. Colditz. 2003. "Relation between Dieting and

Weight Change among Preadolescents and Adolescents." *Pediatrics*, 112: 900–906.

Fikkan, Janna L., and Esther D. Rothblum. 2012. "Is Fat a Feminist Issue? Exploring the Gendered Nature of Weight Bias." *Sex Roles*, 66: 575–92.

Fisancik, Christina. 2009. "Fatness (In)visible: Polycystic Ovarian Syndrome and the Rhetoric of Normative Femininity." In *The Fat Studies Reader*, edited by Esther Rothblum and Sandra Solovay, 106–9. New York: New York University Press.

Flegal, Katherine M., Brian K. Kit, Heather Orpana, and Barry I. Graubard. 2013. "Association of All-Cause Mortality with Overweight and Obesity Using Standard Body Mass Index Categories: A Systematic Review and Meta-Analysis." *JAMA*, 309 (1): 71–82.

Fleischmann, E., N. Teal, J. Dudley, W. May, J. D. Bower, and A. K. Salahudeen. 1999. "Influence of Excess Weight on Mortality and Hospital Stay in 1346 Hemodialysis Patients." *Kidney International*, 55: 1560–67.

Flood, Michael. 2008. "Men, Sex and Homosociality: How Bonds between Men Shape the Sexual Relations with Women." *Men and Masculinities*, 10: 339–59.

Fonarow, G. C., P. Srikanthan, M. R. Costanzo, G. B. Cintron, and M. Lopatin. 2007. "An Obesity Paradox in Acute Heart Failure: Analysis of Body Mass Index and in Hospital Mortality for 108,927 Patients in the Acute Decompensated Heart Failure National Registry." *American Heart Journal*, 153: 74–81.

Foucault, Michel. 1994. *The Birth of the Clinic: An Archaeology of Medical Perception*. New York: Vintage.

———. 1977. *Discipline and Punish: The Birth of the Prison*. New York: Vintage.

Fraser, Laura. 2009. "The Inner Corset: A Brief History of Fat in the United States." In *The Fat Studies Reader*, edited by Esther Rothblum and Sandra Solovay, 11–14. New York: New York University Press.

Freespirit, Judy, and Aldebaran. 2009. "Fat Liberation Manifesto, November 1973." In *The Fat Studies Reader*, edited by Esther Rothblum and Sandra Solovay, 341–42. New York: New York University Press.

Gaesser, Glenn. 2002. *Big Fat Lies*. Carlsbad, CA: Gurze.

Gailey, Jeannine A. Forthcoming. "Transforming the Looking-Glass: Fat Women's Sexual Empowerment through Body Acceptance." In *Fat Sex: New Directions in Theory and Activism*, edited by Helen Hester and Caroline Walters. London: Ashgate.

———. 2012. "Fat Shame to Fat Pride: Fat Women's Sexual and Dating Experiences." *Fat Studies: An Interdisciplinary Journal of Body Weight and Society*, 1 (1): 114–27.

Gailey, Jeannine A., and Ariane Prohaska. 2006. "'Knocking Off a Fat Girl': An Exploration of Hogging, Male Sexuality, and Neutralizations." *Deviant Behavior*, 27: 31–49.

Garland-Thomson, Rosemarie. 2004. "Dares to Stares: Disabled Women Performance Artists and the Dynamics of Staring." In *Bodies in Commotion: Disability and Performance*, edited by P. Auslander and C. Sandahl, 30–42. Ann Arbor: University of Michigan Press.

Garner, D. M., and S. C. Wooley. 1991. "Confronting the Failure of Behavioral and Dietary Treatments for Obesity." *Clinical Psychology Review*, 11: 729–80.

Gecas, V., and P. Burke. 1995. "Self and Identity." In *Sociological Perspectives on Social Psychology*, edited by K. Cook, G. Fine, and J. House, 41–67. Boston: Allyn and Bacon.

Geertz, Clifford. 1973. "Thick Description: Toward an Interpretive Theory of Culture." In *The Interpretation of Cultures: Selected Essays*, 3–30. New York: Basic.

Gimlin, Debra. 2002. *Body Work: Beauty and Self-Image in American Culture*. Berkeley: University of California Press.

Glaser, Barney G., and Anselm L. Strauss. 1967. *The Discovery of Grounded Theory: Strategies for Qualitative Research*. Chicago: Aldine.

Goffman, Erving. 1974. *Frame Analysis: An Essay on the Organization of Experience*. New York: Harper and Row.

———. 1971. *Relations in Public: Microstudies of the Public Order*. New York: Harper and Row.

———. 1963. *Stigma: Notes on the Management of a Spoiled Identity*. Englewood Cliffs, NJ: Prentice-Hall.

Goode, Erich, and Joanne Preissler. 1984. "The Fat Admirer." *Deviant Behavior*, 4: 175–202.

Goran, Michael I., Stanley J. Ulijaszek, and E. Emily Ventura. 2013. "High Fructose Corn Syrup and Diabetes Prevalence: A Global Perspective." *Global Public Health*, 8: 55–64.

Gordon, Avery. 1996. *Ghostly Matter: Haunting and the Sociological Imagination*. Minneapolis: University of Minnesota Press.

Gray, Emma. 2012. "Georgia Anti-Obesity Ads Say 'Stop Sugarcoating' Childhood Obesity." *The Huffington Post*, January 3, 2012: http://www.huffingtonpost.com/2012/01/03/georgia-anti-obesity-ads-stop-sugarcoating_n_1182023.html.

Grosz, Elizabeth. 1994. *Volatile Bodies: Toward a Corporeal Feminism*. Bloomington: Indiana University Press.

Halabi, S., E. J. Small, and N. J. Vogelzang. 2005. "Elevated Body Mass Index Predicts for Longer Overall Survival Duration in Men with Metastatic Hormone Refractory Prostate Cancer." *Journal of Clinical Oncology*, 223: 2434–35.

Haraway, Donna. 2000. "Deanimations: Maps and Portraits of Life Itself." In *Hybridity and Its Discontents: Politics, Science, Culture*, edited by Avtar Brah and Annie E. Coombes, 111–36. New York: Routledge.

Harjunen, Hannele. 2009. *Women and Fat: Approaches to the Social Study of Fatness.* PhD diss., University of Jyväskylä.
Heron, Kristin E., Joshua M. Smyth, Esther Akano, and Stephen A. Wonderlich. 2013. "Assessing Body Image in Young Children: A Preliminary Study of Racial and Developmental Differences." *Sage Open*, 3 (1). Accessed September 13, 2013: doi: 10.1177/2158244013478013
Hesse-Biber, Sharlene Nagy. 2007. *The Cult of Thinness.* New York: Oxford University Press.
Higgins, L. C., and W. Gray. 1998. "Changing the Body Image Concern and Eating Behavior of Chronic Dieters: The Effects of a Psychoeducational Intervention." *Psychology and Health*, 13 (6): 1045–60.
Hoppe, R., and J. Ogden. 1997. "Practice Nurses' Beliefs about Obesity and Weight Related Interventions in Primary Care." *International Journal of Obesity Related Metabolic Disorders*, 21: 141–46.
Huff, Joyce. 2009. "Access to the Sky: Airplane Seats and Fat Bodies as Contested Spaces." In *The Fat Studies Reader*, edited by Esther Rothblum and Sandra Solovay, 176–86. New York: New York University Press.
Huon, G., and J. Lim. 2000. "The Emergence of Dieting among Female Adolescents: Age, Body Mass Index, and Seasonal Effects." *International Journal of Eating Disorders*, 28: 221–25.
Jennings, Laura. 2014. "Visual Representation of Fatness and Health in High School Health Texts." *Fat Studies: An Interdisciplinary Journal of Body Weight and Society*, 3: 45–57.
———. 2010. "Where the [Fat Women's] Bodies Are Buried: A Sociological Look at Women's Clothing Departments." Paper presented at the Popular Culture Association/ACA Annual Meeting, April 2, St. Louis, MO.
Jerant, Anthony, and Peter Franks. 2012. "Body Mass Index, Diabetes, Hypertension, and Short-Term Mortality: A Population Based Observational Study, 2000–2006." *JABFM*, 25 (4): 422–31.
Jersild, A. 1952. *In Search of Self.* New York: Teacher's College Press.
Joanisse, L., and A. Synnott. 1999. "Fighting Back: Reactions and Resistance to the Stigma of Obesity." In *Interpreting Weight: The Social Management of Fatness and Thinness*, edited by J. Sobal and D. Maurer, 49–72. New York: Aldine De Gruyter.
Kalantar-Zadeh, K., K. C. Abbott, A. K. Salahudeen, R. D. Kilpatrick, and T. B. Horwich. 2005. "Survival Advantages of Obesity in Dialysis Patients." *American Journal of Clinical Nutrition*, 81: 543–54.
Katz, Sidney. 2007. "The Importance of Being Beautiful." In *Down to Earth Sociology: Introductory Readings*, 14th edition, edited by James M. Henslin, 341–48. New York: Free Press.
Kent, Le'a. 2001. "Fighting Abjection: Representing Fat Women." In *Bodies Out of Bounds*, edited by Jana Evans Braziel and Kathleen LeBesco, 130–50. Berkeley: University of California Press.

Kirkman, M. Sue, V. J. Briscoe, N. Clark, H. Florez, L. B. Haas, J. B. Halter, E. S. Huang, M. T. Korytkowski, M. N. Munshi, P. S. Odegard, R. E. Pratley, and C. S. Swift. 2012. "Diabetes in Older Adults: A Consensus Report." *Journal of American Geriatrics Society*, 60: 1–15. Accessed on November 16, 2013: doi: 10.1111/jgs.12035

Kitsuse, John I. 1980. "Coming Out All Over: Deviants and the Politics of Social Problems." *Social Problems*, 28: 1–13.

Klein, D., J. Najman, A. F. Kohrman, and C. Munro. 1982. "Patient Characteristics That Elicit Negative Responses from Family Physicians." *Journal of Family Practice*, 14: 881–88.

Koppelman, Susan. 2003. "Afterword." In *The Strange History of Suzanne LaFleshe, and Other Stories of Women and Fatness*, edited by Koppelman, 229–68. New York: Feminist Press at City University of New York.

Krantz, David S., and Melissa K. McCeney. 2002. "Effects of Psychological and Social Factors on Organic Disease: A Critical Assessment of Research on Coronary Heart Disease." *Annual Review of Psychology*, 53: 341–69.

Kristeva, Julia. 1982. *Powers of Horror: An Essay on Abjection*. New York: Columbia University Press.

Kwan, Samantha, and Jennifer Graves. 2013. *Framing Fat*. New Brunswick, NJ: Rutgers University Press.

Kyrölä, Katariina. 2014. *The Weight of Images: Affect, Body Image and Fat in the Media*. London: Ashgate.

———. 2005. "The Fat Gendered Body in/as a Closet." *Feminist Media Studies*, 5: 99–102.

Lainscak, M., S. Haehling, W. Doehner, and S. D. Anker. 2012. "The Obesity Paradox in Chronic Disease: Facts and Numbers." *Journal of Cachex Sarcopenia Muscle*, 3: 1–4.

Lamarche, B., J. P. Després, M. C. Pouliot, S. Moorjani, P. J. Lupien, G. Thériault, A. Tremblay, A. Nadeau, and C. Bouchard. 1992. "Is Body Fat Loss a Determinant Factor in the Improvement of Carbohydrate and Lipid Metabolism following Aerobic Exercise Training in Obese Women?" *Metabolism*, 41: 1249–56.

LeBesco, Kathleen. 2004. *Revolting Bodies? The Struggle to Redefine Fat Identity*. Amherst: University of Massachusetts Press.

———. 2001. "Queering Fat Bodies/Politics." In *Bodies Out of Bounds*, edited by Jana Evans Braziel and Kathleen LeBesco, 74–87. Berkeley: University of California Press.

Lepoff, Laurie Ann. 1983. "Fat Politics." In *Shadow on a Tightrope: Writings by Women on Fat Oppression*, edited by Lisa Schoenfielder and Barb Wieser, 204–9. Iowa City, IA: Aunt Lute.

Lewis, D. M., and F. M. Cachelin. 2001. "Body Image, Body Dissatisfaction, and Eating Attitudes in Midlife and Elderly Women." *Eating Disorders*, 9 (1): 29–39.

Lupton, Deborah. 2012. *Fat*. New York: Routledge.

Lustig, Robert H. 2013. *Fat Chance: Beating the Odds against Sugar, Processed Food, Obesity, and Disease.* New York: Plume.

Lyons, Pat. 2009. "Prescription for Harm: Diet Industry Influence, Public Health Policy, and the 'Obesity Epidemic.'" In *The Fat Studies Reader*, edited by Esther Rothblum and Sandra Solovay, 75–87. New York: New York University Press.

Maiman, L. A., V. L. Wang, M. H. Becker, J. Finlay, and M. Simonson. 1979. "Attitudes toward Obesity and the Obese among Professionals." *Journal of American Dietetic Association*, 74: 331–36.

Mann, T., A. J. Tomiyama, E. Westling, A. M. Lew, B. Samuels, and J. Chatman. 2007. "Medicare's Search for Effective Obesity Treatments: Diets Are Not the Answer." *American Psychologist*, 62 (3): 220–33.

Maroney, D., and S. Golub. 1992. "Nurses' Attitudes toward Obese Persons and Certain Ethnic Groups." *Perception and Motor Skills*, 75: 387–91.

Mason, Katherine. 2012. "The Unequal Weight of Discrimination: Gender, Body Size, and Income Inequality." *Social Problems*, 59 (3): 411–35.

McEvoy, Sharlene A. 1992. "Fat Chance: Employment Discrimination against the Overweight." *Labor Law Journal*, 43 (1): 3–14.

Mead, George H. [1934] 1967. *Mind, Self, and Society: From the Standpoint of a Social Behaviorist.* Chicago: University of Chicago Press.

Miller, Wayne C. 1999. "Fitness and Fatness in Relation to Health: Implications for a Paradigm Shift." *Journal of Social Issues*, 55 (2): 207–19.

Millman, Marcia. 1980. *Such a Pretty Face: Being Fat in America.* New York: W. W. Norton.

Mitchell, Allyson. 2005. "Pissed Off." In *Fat: The Anthropology of Obsession*, edited by Don Kulick and Anne Meneley, 211–25. New York: Tarcher/Penguin.

Muennig, Peter. 2008. "The Body Politic: The Relationship between Stigma and Obesity-Associated Disease." *BioMed Central Public Health*, 8: 128–38.

Murray, Samantha. 2008. *The Fat Female Body.* Basingstoke, England: Palgrave Macmillan.

———. 2005. "(Un/be) Coming Out? Rethinking Fat Politics." *Social Semiotics*, 15: 153–63.

———. 2004. "Locating Aesthetics: Sexing the Fat Woman." *Social Semiotics*, 14: 237–47.

Neumark-Sztainer, D., M. Wall, J. Guo, M. Story, J. Haines, and M. Eisenberg. 2006. "Obesity, Disordered Eating, and Eating Disorders in a Longitudinal Study of Adolescents: How Do Dieters Fare 5 Years Later?" *Journal of the American Dietetics Association*, 106: 559–68.

Neumark-Sztainer, D., Melanie Wall, Mary Story, and Amber R. Standish. 2012. "Dieting and Unhealthy Weight Control Behaviors during Adolescence: Associations with 10-Year Changes in Body Mass Index." *Journal of Adolescent Health*, 50 (1): 80–86.

Newmahr, Staci. 2011. *Playing on the Edge: Sadomasochism, Risk, and Intimacy.* Bloomington: Indiana University Press.

Oakley, A. 1981. "Interviewing Women: A Contradiction in Terms." In *Doing Feminist Research*, edited by H. Roberts, 147–61. London: Heinemann.

Oldroyd, J., M. Banerjee, A. Heald, and K. Cruickshank. 2005. "Diabetes and Ethnic Minorities." *Postgraduate Medical Journal*, 81: 486–90. Accessed on November 16, 2013: doi: 10.1136/pgmj.2004.029124

Oliver, J. Eric. 2006. *Fat Politics: The Real Story behind America's Obesity Epidemic.* New York: Oxford University Press.

Orbach, Susie. 1978. *Fat Is a Feminist Issue: The Anti-Diet Guide to Permanent Weight Loss.* London: Arrow.

Ortega, F. B., D. C. Lee, P. T. Katzmarzyk, J. R. Ruiz, X. Sui, T. S. Church, and S. N. Blair. 2012. "The Intriguing Metabolically Healthy but Obese Phenotype: Cardiovascular Prognosis and Role of Fitness." *European Heart Journal*, 34 (5): 389–97. Accessed on November 15, 2013: doi:10.1093/eurheartj/ehs174

Owen, Lesleigh. 2012. "Living Fat in a Thin-Centric World: Effects of Spatial Discrimination on Fat Bodies and Selves." *Feminism & Psychology*, 22 (3): 290–306.

Patsa, C., K. Toutouzas, E. Tsiamis, C. Tsioufis, A. Spanos, A. Karanasos, A. Michelongona, D. Tousoulis, and C. Stefanadis. 2013. "Impact of Metabolic Syndrome on Clinical Outcomes after New Generation Drug-Eluting Stent Implantation: The 'Obesity Paradox' Phenomenon Is Still Apparent." *Nutrition, Metabolism, and Cardiovascular Diseases*, 4: 307–13.

Patton, G. C., R. Selzer, C. Coffey, J. B. Carlin, and R. Wolfe. 1999. "Onset of Adolescent Eating Disorders: Population Based Cohort Study over 3 Years." *British Medical Journal*, 318: 765–68.

Perez, Marisol, and Thomas E. Joiner Jr. 2003. "Body Image Dissatisfaction and Disordered Eating in Black and White Women." *Internal Journal of Eating Disorders*, 33 (3): 342–50.

Pingitore, A., G. Di Bella, M. Lombardi, G. Iervasi, E. Strata, G. D. Aquaro, V. Positano, D. De Marchi, G. Rossi, A. L'Abbate, and D. Rovai. 2007. "The Obesity Paradox and Myocardial Infarct Size." *Journal of Cardiovascular Medicine*, 8: 713–17.

Pitts, Victoria. 2003. *In the Flesh: The Cultural Politics of Body Modification.* New York: Palgrave Macmillan.

Price, J. H., S. M. Desmond, R. A. Krol, F. F. Snyder, and J. K. O'Connell. 1987. "Family Practice Physicians' Beliefs, Attitudes, and Practices Regarding Obesity." *American Journal of Preventive Medicine*, 3: 339–45.

Prohaska, Ariane, and Jeannine A. Gailey. 2010. "Achieving Masculinity through Sexual Predation: The Case of Hogging." *Journal of Gender Studies*, 19 (1): 13–25.

———. 2009. "Fat Women as 'Easy Targets': Achieving Masculinity through Hogging." In *The Fat Studies Reader*, edited by Esther Rothblum and Sandra Solovay, 158–66. New York: New York University Press.

Puhl, Rebecca M., and Chelsea A. Heuer. 2010. "Obesity Stigma: Important Considerations for Public Health." *American Journal of Public Health*, 100: 1019–28.

Puhl, Rebecca M., Jaime Lee Peterson, and Joerg Luedicke. 2012. "Strategies to Address Weight-Based Victimization: Youths' Preferred Support Intervention from Classmates, Teachers, and Parents." *Journal of Youth Adolescence*, 42 (3): 315–27. Accessed on February 13, 2013: doi: 10.1007/s10964-012-9849-5

Rajaram, Prem Kumar, and Carl Grundy-Warr. 2004. "The Irregular Migrant as *Homo Sacer*: Migration and Detention in Australia, Malaysia, and Thailand." *International Migration*, 42: 33–64.

Rand, C. S., and A. M. MacGregor. 1990. "Morbidly Obese Patients' Perceptions of Social Discrimination before and after Surgery for Obesity." *South Medical Journal*, 83 (12): 1390–95.

Reas, Deborah L., and Carlos M. Grilo. 2007. "Timing and Sequence of the Onset of Overweight, Dieting, and Binge Eating in Overweight Patients with Binge Eating Disorder." *International Journal of Eating Disorders*, 40: 165–70.

Rebelos, E., E. Muscelli, A. Natali, B. Balkau, G. Mingrone, P. Piatti, T. Konrad, A. Mari, and E. Ferrannini. 2011. "Body Weight, Not Insulin Sensitivity or Secretion, May Predict Spontaneous Weight Changes in Nondiabetic and Prediabetic Subjects." *Diabetes*, 60 (7): 1938–45.

Register, C., and D. Williams. 1990. "Wage Effects of Obesity among Young Workers." *Social Science Quarterly*, 71 (1): 130–41.

Rhode, Deborah L. 2010. *The Beauty Bias: The Injustice of Appearance in Life and Law*. New York: Oxford University Press.

Rodin, J., L. R. Silberstein, and R. H. Striegel-Moore. 1985. "Women and Weight: A Normative Discontent." In *Nebraska Symposium on Motivation*, edited by R. Sonderegger, 267–307. Lincoln: University of Nebraska Press.

Rose, Nikolas S. 1999. *Powers of Freedom: Reframing Political Thought*. New York: Cambridge University Press.

Rothblum, Esther D., Pamela A. Brand, Carol T. Miller, and Helen A. Oetjen. 1990. "The Relationship between Obesity, Employment Discrimination, and Employment-Related Victimization." *Journal of Vocational Behavior*, 37: 251–66.

Rothblum, Esther D., and Sondra Solovay. 2009. *The Fat Studies Reader*. New York: New York University Press.

Royce, Tracy. 2009. "The Shape of Abuse: Fat Oppression as a Form of Violence against Women." In *The Fat Studies Reader*, edited by Esther Rothblum and Sandra Solovay, 151–57. New York: New York University Press.

Saguy, Abigail C. 2013. *What's Wrong with Fat?* New York: Oxford University Press.

Saguy, Abigail C., and Kjerstin Gruys. 2010. "Morality and Health: News Media Contructions of Overweight and Eating Disorders." *Social Problems*, 57 (2): 231–50.

Saguy, Abigail C., and Kevin W. Riley. 2005. "Weighing Both Sides: Morality, Mortality, and Framing Contests over Obesity." *Journal of Health Politics, Policy and Law*, 30: 869–921.

Saguy, Abigail C., and Anna Ward. 2011. "Coming Out as Fat: Rethinking Stigma." *Social Psychology Quarterly*, 74 (1): 53–75.

Sanchez, Diana T., and Amy K. Kiefer. 2007. "Body Concerns in and out of the Bedroom: Implications for Sexual Pleasure and Problems." *Archives of Sexual Behavior*, 36: 808–20.

Sartore, M., and G. Cunningham. 2007. "Weight Discrimination, Hiring Recommendations, Person-Job Fit, and Attributes: Fitness Industry Implications." *Journal of Sport Management*, 21 (2): 172–93.

Schallenkamp, Ken, Ron DeBeaumont, and Joshua Houy. 2012. "Weight-Based Discrimination in the Workplace: Is Legal Protection Necessary?" *Employee Responsibility & Rights Journal*, 24: 251–59.

Schur, Edwin. 1984. *Labeling Women Deviant: Gender, Stigma, and Social Control*. New York: Random House.

Schvey, Natasha A., Rebecca M. Puhl, and Kelly D. Brownell. 2014. "The Stress of Stigma: Exploring the Effect of Weight Stigma on Cortisol Reactivity." *Psychosomatic Medicine*, 76: published ahead of print 0.1097/ PSY.0000000000000031. Accessed April 5, 2014.

Schwartz, M. B., H. O'Neal, K. D. Brownell, S. Blair, and C. Billington. 2003. "Weight Bias among Health Professionals Specializing in Obesity." *Obesity Research*, 11: 1033–39.

Schwartz, Marlene B., Lenny R. Vartanian, Brian A. Nosek, and Kelly D. Brownell. 2006. "The Influence of One's Own Body Weight on Implicit and Explicit Anti-Fat Bias." *Obesity*, 14: 440–47.

Sedgwick, Eve Kosofsky. 2000. *A Dialogue on Love*. Boston, MA: Beacon.

———. 1993. *Tendencies*. Durham, NC: Duke University Press.

———. 1990. *Epistemology of the Closet*. Berkeley: University of California Press.

Serpe, Richard T., and Sheldon Stryker. 1987. "The Construction of Self and Reconstruction of Social Relationships." In *Advances in Group Process*, edited by E. Lawler and B. Markovsky, 41–66. Greenwich, CT: JAI.

Silber, T. J. 1986. "Anorexia Nervosa in Blacks and Hispanics." *International Journal of Eating Disorders*, 5 (1): 121–28.

Sinding, C., and J. Aronson. 2003. "Exposing Failures, Unsettling Accommodations: Tensions in Interview Practice." *Qualitative Research*, 3 (1): 95–117.

Sorensen, T. I. A. 1995. "Socio-Economic Aspects of Obesity: Causes or Effects." *International Journal of Obesity*, 19: S6–S8.

Squires, Sally. 1998. "Optimal Weight Threshold Lowered: Millions More to Be Termed Overweight." *Washington Post*, June 4.

Star, Susan Leigh, and Anselm Strauss. 1999. "Layers of Silence, Arenas of Voice: The Ecology of Visible and Invisible Work." *Computer Supported Cooperative Work*, 8: 9–30.

Stone, Gregory P. 1962. "Appearance and the Self." In *Human Behavior and Social Processes: An Interactionist Approach*, edited by Arnold Rose, 86–116. Boston: Houghton Mifflin.

Storz, N., and W. Greene. 1983. "Body Weight, Body Image, and Perception of Fad Diets in Adolescent Girls." *Journal of Nutritional Education*, 15: 15–18.

Stryker, Sheldon. 2000. "Identity Competition: Key to Differential Social Movement Involvement." In *Identity, Self, and Social Movements*, edited by S. Stryker, T. Owens, and R. White, 21–40. Minneapolis: University of Minnesota Press.

———. 1980. *Symbolic Interactionism: A Social Structural Version*. Menlo Park, CA: Benjamin Cummings.

———. 1968. "Identity Salience and Role Performance." *Journal of Marriage and the Family*, 4: 558–64.

Stryker, Sheldon, and Richard T. Serpe. 1994. "Identity Salience and Psychological Centrality: Equivalent, Overlapping, or Complementary Concepts?" *Social Psychology Quarterly*, 57: 16–35.

———. 1982. "Commitment, Identity Salience, and Role Behavior: A Theory and Research Example." In *Personality, Roles, and Social Behavior*, edited by W. Ickes and E. S. Knowles, 199–218. New York: Springer-Verlag.

Stunkard, Albert J., and Kelly Costello Allison. 2003. "Two Forms of Disordered Eating in Obesity: Binge Eating and Night Eating." *International Journal of Obesity*, 27: 1–12.

Sutin, Angelina R., and Antonio Terracciano. 2013. "Perceived Weight Discrimination and Obesity." *PLoS ONE* 8 (7): e70048. Accessed July 25, 2013: doi: 10.1371/journal.pone.0070048

Swami, Viren, and Martin J. Tovèe. 2009. "Big Beautiful Women: The Body Size Preferences of Male Fat Admirers." *Journal of Sex Research*, 46: 89–96.

Teachman, B. A., and K. D. Brownell. 2001. "Implicit Anti-Fat Bias among Health Professionals: Is Anyone Immune?" *International Journal of Obesity and Related Metabolic Disorders: Journal of the International Association for the Study of Obesity*, 25 (10): 1525–31.

Teegardin, Carrie. 2012. "Grim Childhood Obesity Ads Stir Critics." *The Atlanta Journal Constitution*, January 1, 2012.

thunder. 1983. "Coming Out: Notes of Fat Lesbian Pride." In *Shadow on a Tightrope: Writings by Women on Fat Oppression*, edited by Lisa Schoenfielder and Barb Wieser, 210–15. Iowa City, IA: Aunt Lute.

Tischner, Irmgard. 2013. *Fat Lives: A Feminist Psychological Exploration*. New York: Routledge.

Tischner, Irmgard, and Helen Malson. 2012. "Deconstructing Health and the Un/healthy 'Fat' Woman." *Journal of Community and Applied Social Psychology*, 22 (1): 50–62.

———. 2008. "Exploring the Politics of Women's In/Visible 'Large' Bodies." *Feminism and Psychology*, 18 (2): 260–67.

Tovar, Virgie. 2012. *Hot and Heavy: Fierce Fat Girls on Life, Love, and Fashion*. Berkeley, CA: Seal.

Trogdon, J. G., E. A. Finkelstein, T. Hylands, P. S. Dellea, and S. J. Kamal-Bahl. 2008. "Indirect Costs of Obesity: A Review of the Current Literature." *Obesity Review*, 9: 489–500.

Veblen, Thorstein. [1899] 1994. *Theory of the Leisure Class*. Reprint Edition. New York: Dover.

Wann, Marilyn. 2009. "Forward: Fat Studies: An Invitation to Revolution." In *The Fat Studies Reader*, edited by Esther Rothblum and Sandra Solovay, ix–xxv. New York: New York University Press.

———. 1998. *Fat!So?* Berkeley, CA: Ten Speed.

Waskul, Dennis D., and Phillip Vannini. 2006. "Introduction: The Body in Symbolic Interaction." In *Body/Embodiment: Symbolic Interaction and the Sociology of the Body*, edited by Dennis Waskul and Phillip Vannini, 1–18. Burlington, VT: Ashgate.

Weinstein, Rebecca. 2012. *Fat Sex: The Naked Truth*. Self-published.

West, Candace, and Sarah Fenstermaker. 1995. "Doing Difference." *Gender & Society*, 9 (1): 8–37.

West, Candace, and Don H. Zimmerman. 1987. "Doing Gender." *Gender & Society*, 1 (2): 125–51.

Wheeler, L., and Y. Kim. 1997. "What Is Beautiful Is Culturally Good: The Physical Attractiveness Stereotype Has Different Content in Collectivist Cultures." *Personality and Social Psychology Bulletin*, 23: 795–800.

Wiederman, Michael W., and Shannon R. Hurst. 2008. "Body Size, Physical Attractiveness, and Body Image among Young Adult Women: Relationships to Sexual Experience and Sexual Esteem." *Journal of Sex Research*, 35: 272–81.

Wolf, Naomi. [1991] 2002. *The Beauty Myth: How Images of Beauty Are Used against Women*. New York: Harper Perennial.

Yanovski, S. Z. 2003. "Binge Eating Disorder and Obesity in 2003: Could Treating an Eating Disorder Have a Positive Effect on the Obesity Epidemic?" *International Journal of Eating Disorders*, 34: S117–S120.

Young, L. M., and B. Powell. 1985. "The Effects of Obesity on the Clinical Judgments of Mental Health Professionals." *Journal of Health and Social Behavior*, 26: 233–46.

Zitzelsberger, Hilde. 2005. "(In)visibility: Accounts of Embodiment of Women with Physical Disabilities and Differences." *Disability & Society*, 20: 389–403.

Index

abjection, 57, 79–80
abuse. *See* mistreatment and abuse
activism. *See* fat activism and activists; size acceptance movement
Adipositivity Project, 150–51
African Americans, 32, 124, 159–62
age and confidence, 132, 142
alcoholism, medicalization of, 84
Aldebaran, 26
Alexander, C. Normal, 34
Allison, Kelly Costello, 74
alternate sexual lifestyles, 126–28, 168
American Medical Association (AMA), 83, 109
American Psychiatric Association (APA), 70
American Sociological Association (ASA), 166
amphetamines, 61, 81, 184n2
Amy, Nancy K., 3, 94
Andreyeva, Tatiana, 15
anorexia, 15, 70–72, 79, 141, 152
anxiety, 49, 81, 84, 86, 99, 146
appearance: self-esteem and self-value tied to, 51–54, 55, 82; visibility spectrum and, 8–12
Armstrong, D., 87
Aronson, J., 180
asexuality, 28, 111, 112, 117, 133–34, 170
Averett, Susan, 3, 171

Bacon, Linda, 86, 105, 106
Bagley, C. R., 85
Banerjee, M., 22
Baum, Charles, 171
BDSM (bondage, discipline, sadomasochism), 127
Beauboeuf-Lafontant, Tamara, 32
Beauty Myth, The (Wolf), 53
beauty standards: in Brazilian culture, 64; in Dominican Republic, 62; fat/bad and thin/good dichotomy, 112–13, 137–38, 157–58; gender roles and, 53, 187n1; ideal female bodies, 79–80, 133, 138–39; in lesbian communities, 126; media fueling, 137; men and beauty standards, 187n1; myth of beauty, 53; sexuality and social norms of, 111–15, 133; social surveillance and policing, 57, 61–65; thin privilege, 3, 10–11, 39–40, 59, 137–38. *See also* thinness
Becker, M., 87
BED (binge eating disorder), 1, 63, 70, 71, 74–75, 78, 150
BEDA (Binge Eating Disorder Association), 101
Bentham, Jeremy, 10
Berg, Frances M., 73, 150
Big Beautiful Women (BBW), 26, 146, 156

Big Big Love (Blank), 186n1
Biggest Loser, The (TV show), 19–20, 23
binge eating disorder (BED), 1, 63, 70, 71, 74–75, 78, 150
Binge Eating Disorder Association (BEDA), 101
Bjorntorp, P., 103
Black Feminist Thought (Collins), 161–62
Blank, Hanne, 186n1
blogs, 85–86, 139, 157
Blumberg, P., 85
BMI. *See* body mass index (BMI)
bodies, social control of: body/mind separation, 42, 52–58, 66–67, 129, 142; body shame and sexuality, 5, 117–23; corsets, 2–3, 35–37, 55, 81, 113, 117–23, 134; fear of fat, 37–38, 44–45, 55, 57, 114–16, 117; fixing bodies, societal focus on, 57–65, 81; social surveillance and policing, 10, 35–40, 51, 59, 62–64, 113; visibility as control, 18–19
body acceptance: age and confidence, 132, 142; beauty standards and, 6, 138–39; diversity in body types and, 170; embodiment of fat, 133, 141, 143–47, 149, 158–59; sexual enjoyment and, 126
body image, shifting views on, 126–35
body mass index (BMI): cancer screening tests and, 94; categories, 20–21, 154; changing categories, 21, 154; dieting and, 81; disease label of obesity and, 83; focus on *vs.* on health, 75; normal, 20; "obese" category, 20, 40, 154; overweight, 20–21; problems in calculating, 21; recommendations on, 73
body/mind separation, 42, 52–58, 66–67, 129, 142
Bodypositive.com, 163
body shame, 117–23
body size and genetics, 3, 21, 60, 149–50
Boero, Natalie, 4, 15, 21, 32, 42, 55, 83, 87, 111, 113, 165
Bordo, Susan, 113, 137
Boston Medical Center, 65
Bouchard, C., 149
Braziel, Jana Evans, 112
Brazil, beauty standards in, 64
breast cancer, 18, 89
Brighenti, Andrea, 9, 18–19, 167
Brittingham, Kim, 44–45
Brownell, Kelly D., 3, 15, 24, 97, 165, 171
bulimia, 70–72, 152
bullying: from family, 40–41; fatphobia and, 37–41; in gyms, 37, 69–70; self-esteem, effect on, 38–39
Burgard, Deb, 21, 86, 90, 106, 107
Burke, P., 34
Butler, Judith, 7, 57, 156

Cachelin, F. M., 137
Cahnman, Werner J., 31, 183n4
caloric restriction, 65–66, 68–69, 70–74
Campos, Paul, 21, 22, 88, 97, 103, 149, 150, 164
Camus, Albert, 185n11
cancer: breast cancer, 18, 89; colon cancer, 159–60; fat as protection from, 103; gynecological cancers, 94; uterine cancer, 94
Cao, Sissi, 88
capitalism and diet culture, 67–68
cardiovascular disease, 22, 70, 91, 93
Casper, Monica J., 6–7, 19, 165, 171

Cassuto, J., 103
Cawley, J., 87, 171
CDC (Centers for Disease Control and Prevention), 20, 21, 23–24, 87
Centers for Disease Control and Prevention (CDC), 20, 21, 23–24, 87
Chastain, Ragen, 85–86, 164
childhood obesity, 41, 55, 57, 61–62, 83–84, 184n7
cholesterol, 21, 80–81, 103, 104
Christie, Chris, 15
civil rights, 25, 140
class status. *See* socioeconomic status
clothing sizes, 8–9, 25, 27, 70, 152
Cogan, Jeanine C., 70, 88, 97, 150
Colberg, Sheri R., 22
collective knowingness, 31, 60
college campuses, 45
Collins, Patricia Hill, 161–62
colon cancer, 159–60
coming out as fat, 35–37, 142–43, 154, 159
confidence. *See* body acceptance; self-acceptance; self-esteem
Connell, R. W., 111–12
Conrad, Peter, 84, 87
consumerism: diet industry and diet culture, 21, 24, 67–68, 74, 81–82; focus on thinness, 39
control. *See* bodies, social control of; discipline and control
Cooley, Charles Horton, 15, 41
Cooper, Charlotte, 25–26, 27, 31, 142–43, 150
corsets, 2–3
courtesy stigma, 114, 115, 118
"covering" concept, 50, 143
Crandall, C. S., 44
Crawford, Robert, 87
Critical Weight Studies. *See* Fat Studies
Crosnoe, Robert, 3, 171
Cross, W. E., Jr., 42

Cruickshank, K., 22
Cunningham, G., 171

Dances with Fat (blog), 85–86, 164
Darby, Anita, Phillipa Hay, 3, 170
dating and relationships: abusive relationships, feelings of deserving, 47–48, 50, 55–56, 117–23, 134–35; BBW (Big Beautiful Women) groups, 26, 146, 156; body shame and, 5, 117–23; fat admirers, 5, 26, 114, 124; fat hatred and gender roles, 123–26; loving partners, 130–32; men in control of, 125; mistreatment, fears of, 114–16, 124–25; mistreatment by partners, 43–44, 118–19; online dating, 121, 125; other's perceptions of fat and, 47–48, 50–51, 55, 123–26; same-sex relationships, 125–26
DeAngelis, Tory, 32
death, weight stigma causing, 83–84, 101–2
DeBeaumont, Ron, 171
Denzin, Norman K., 179
depression, 56, 77, 81, 88; anxiety, 49, 81, 84, 86, 99, 146; suicide, 39, 56, 163, 168
diabetes: as assumed health risk for fat persons, 1, 21–23, 92, 98, 104; hyper(in)visibility and, 68; medication used for weight loss, 65–66; Type 1 diabetes, 83–84; Type 2 diabetes, 21–22, 65–66, 83–84; weight gain and, 21–23
Diagnostic Statistical Manual of Mental Disorders (DSM-V), 70
diet culture, 65–70, 81–82; consumerism and, 67–68, 81–82
diet industry, 21, 24, 67–68, 74, 81–82

dieting: about, 65, 70; difficulties in maintaining, 65–67; exercise and, 69–70; extreme diets, 73, 76; food and caloric restriction, 65–66, 68–69, 70–74; hCG diet, 73; healthful eating *vs.*, 28, 79–81, 90, 155–56, 185n10; "normal" size ideals, 81–82; physician-monitored diets, 73, 76; regaining weight, 57, 65–67, 73–74; risks of, 70; types of, 65; Very Low Calorie Diets (VLCD), 73; weight cycling, 22, 65, 73–74, 80, 88–89, 179; work-related diets, 68–69. *See also* eating disorders; weight loss

diet pills, 21, 65–66, 81–82, 85

diets: fasting diets, 62; liquid diets, 80

Dion, Karen, 138

disabled people, visibility and, 10, 11–12

discipline and control: eating disorders and, 79–80; fat as lazy stereotype *vs.*, 19–20, 31, 38–39, 44, 55–56, 66–67, 97, 134; fear of fat as contagious and, 37–38, 44–45, 55, 57, 114–16, 117, 124–25; social surveillance and policing, 10, 35–40, 51, 59, 62–64, 113; thinness as symbol of, 39–40, 71

discrediting attributes, 24, 31, 147

discrimination: bullying and fatphobia, 37–41, 69–70; feelings of deserving, 47, 48, 50, 55–56, 117–23, 134–35; internalizing fat hatred and, 41–47, 54–55, 56, 57, 117; laws against, 170–71; media emphasis on health and, 41, 42–43, 55; microaggressions, 49–50, 99; social surveillance and policing, 10, 35–40, 51, 59, 62–64, 113; spatial discrimination, 49–51; weight discrimination, laws on, 170–71

disease label. *See* obesity as epidemic/disease

disordered eating (EDNOS), 70–76. *See also* eating disorders

doctors, avoiding, 22, 84–86, 88, 97–102

"doing difference" concept, 47

"doing fat" concept: about, 16–17, 47–48; as activism, 150–53, 159; coming out as fat, 35–37, 142–43, 154, 159; gender roles and, 123–26; internalizing fat hatred and, 47; limitations of, 156–57; other's perceptions of fat and, 47–48, 50–51, 55, 123–26; visibility spectrum and, 168

"doing gender" concept, 16–17, 47, 123, 126

Dolezal, Luna, 10–11

Dominican Republic, beauty standards in, 62

Dooley-Hash, Suzanne, 101–2

dumping syndrome, 77–78

eating disorders: about, 70–71; anorexia, 15, 70–72, 79, 141, 152; binge eating disorder (BED), 1, 63, 70, 71, 74–75, 78, 150; bulimia, 70–72, 152; dieting and, 70; disordered exercise, 70, 71–72, 74; EDNOS (eating disorders not otherwise specified), 70, 71, 72; food and caloric restriction, 65–66, 68–69, 70–74; health risks, 70; physician-monitored diets and, 73, 76

eating habits: diet culture and, 67–69; healthful eating, 28, 79–81, 90, 155–56, 185n10; modifying for weight loss, 45

Edleman, Marian Wright, 170
EDNOS (eating disorders not otherwise specified), 70, 71, 72
emphasized femininity, 111–12
employee wellness programs, 68–69
epidemics: defined, 3–4; postmodern epidemics, 4. *See also* obesity as epidemic/disease
Ernsberger, Paul, 3, 21, 22, 24, 88, 97, 171
exercise: diabetes and, 21–22; dieting and, 69–70; disordered eating and, 70, 71; disordered exercise, 70, 71–72, 74; motivations for, 1, 45, 69, 93, 96; in public spaces, 37, 45–46, 69–70
extreme diets, 73, 76

Fabrey, William, 25, 139
failing, feelings of, 33, 38–39, 42–43, 46–48, 126–27, 158, 161–62
family: bullying and harassment from, 40–41, 43; pressure to fix fat bodies from, 1, 43, 57, 59–61, 95–97; women's roles in, 87–88
Farrell, Amy, 24, 31, 117, 148, 164
fast food, 155, 185n10
fasting, 74
fasting diets, 62
fat, becoming, 33
fat, usage of word, 2, 3, 4, 140–41, 152, 158
fat acceptance movement. *See* size acceptance movement
fat activism and activists: about, 26–27, 84–86, 143–44, 147, 150–53; Adipositivity Project, 150–51; Chastain, Ragen, 85–86, 164; Cooper, Charlotte, 25–26, 27, 31, 142–43, 150; "doing fat" as activism, 150–53; Health at Every Size (HAES), 28, 54, 80, 86, 105–7, 155, 169; Jones, Substantia, 150–51; Mitchell, Allyson, 151–52; Oelbaum, Brenda, 152; in online communities, 139–40; Pretty Porky and Pissed Off, 151–52, 159; Wann, Marilyn, 3, 20, 26, 31, 84–85, 108, 143, 144, 151. *See also* size acceptance movement
fat activism via: online communities, 139–40
fat admirers, 5, 26, 114, 124
Fat and Proud (Cooper), 26
fat/bad and thin/good dichotomy, 112–13, 137–38, 157–58
"fat drag," 151
"Fat Enough to Belong" (blog), 157
Fat Female Body, The (Murray), 3–4, 154
fat fetishists. *See* fat admirers
"fat girl mentality," 51, 56
fat hatred: antifat attitudes from fat persons, 44–45; fear of fat, 37–38, 44–45, 55, 57, 114–16, 117; hyper(in)visibility and, 12–19; judgment and other's perceptions, 45–47; media emphasis on health and, 41, 42–43, 55
fat hatred, internalization of: abjection and, 57, 79–80
fat identity, embodiment of, 133, 141, 143–47, 149, 158–59. *See also* body acceptance; self identity
Fat Industrial Complex, 24
Fat Is a Feminist Issue (Orbach), 113
Fat Liberation Manifesto, 25–26
fat-o-sphere, 26, 139–40, 141, 143–44, 159
fatphobia: about, 33, 85; bullying and, 37–41, 69–70; effect

fatphobia (*continued*)
  of, 15, 85; fear of fat, 37–38, 44–45, 55, 57, 114–16, 117; hyper(in)visibility and, 15, 38, 150–51
Fat Politics (Oliver), 21
fat pride. *See* body acceptance; self-acceptance; size acceptance movement
Fat Sex (Weinstein), 27, 186n1
Fat Shame (Farrell), 164
Fat!So? (Wann), 26, 144
Fat Studies: about, 3; growth of research on, 165–66; on obesity as epidemic, 3, 84–86; size acceptance movement, 26
Fat Studies: An Interdisciplinary Journal of Body Weight and Society, 26, 126, 135, 166
Fat Studies Reader, The, 26, 166
Fat Underground (FU), 25–26
fear of fat, 37–38, 44–45, 55, 57, 114–16, 117
femininity: "doing fat" and gender roles, 123–26; gender-roles norms and, 80, 111–12, 115, 132–33
feminism: eating disorders and, 15; Fat Studies in, 166; humanism *vs.*, 187n5; humanist *vs.* feminist, 187n5
Fenske, Sarah, 4, 5
Fenstermaker, Sarah, 47
Field, A. E., 67, 71, 75
Fikkan, Janna L., 15, 25
Fisancik, Christina, 93
flaunting, 143, 151, 152
Fleischmann, E., 102–3
Flood, Michael, 115
Fonarow, G., 103
food: caloric restriction and, 65–66, 68–69, 70–74; diet culture and, 67–70; fast food, 155, 185n10; industrialization and, 39; junk food, 22, 106–7, 155, 185; relationship with, 51, 106–7
food restriction, 65–66, 68–69, 70–74
foot binding, 64–65
Ford, William, 171
Foucault, Michel, 9–10, 19, 79, 87, 162, 167
framing, 112–13
Franks, Peter, 22
Fraser, Laura, 39
Freespirit, Judy, 26

Gailey, Jeannine A., 5, 35, 111–15, 126, 127, 133, 135, 142, 156, 173, 175, 176
Garland-Thomson, Rosemarie, 11, 167
Garner, D. M., 22, 88, 150
gastric banding (lap band surgery), 2, 39–40, 61, 76, 184n3
gastric bypass surgery, 2, 76–77, 78, 89
Gecas, V., 34
Geertz, Clifford, 173
gender: "doing fat" and gender roles, 123–26; "doing gender" concept, 16–17, 47, 123, 126; emphasized femininity, 111–12; family roles for women, 87–88; fat as both masculine and feminine, 80, 111–12, 115, 132–33; hegemonic masculinity, 80, 111–12, 115; men and beauty standards, 187n1
gender roles: body size and social views on, 111–14, 135
generalized other, 34
genetics and obesity, 3, 21, 60, 149–50
Georgia, 41, 55, 184n7
Gimlin, Debra, 5
Glaser, Barney G., 169, 178
"globesity," 88

Goffman, Erving, 11, 24, 25, 31, 35, 50, 82, 112, 114, 143, 148, 1115
Golub, S., 85
Goode, Erich, 5, 114
Goran, Michael I., 22
Graves, Jennifer, 14, 32, 87
Gray, W., 65
Greene, W., 65
Grilo, Carlos M., 75
grocery stores, fatphobia in, 38, 58–59
Grosz, Elizabeth, 79
Grundy-Warr, Carl, 11
Gruys, Kjerstin, 71
gyms, challenges in, 37, 45–46, 69–70
gynecological cancers, 94

HAES (Health at Every Size), 28, 54, 80, 86, 105–7, 155, 169
Halabi, S., 103
Haraway, Donna, 179
Harjunen, Hannele, 84, 183n1
Haskew, P., 22, 88
HBO, 19, 24
hCG diet, 73
Heald, A., 22
health, emphasis on. *See* neoliberalism; obesity as epidemic/disease
health ailments: cardiovascular disease, 22, 70, 91, 93; high blood pressure, 1, 23, 80, 89, 103; hypertension, 21, 23, 56; hypothyroidism, 60, 91, 93, 163; lipedema, 94–95, 163; mobility problems, 38, 59, 155; polycystic ovarian syndrome (PCOS), 40, 60, 93, 163, 184n6
Health at Every Size (Bacon), 105
Health at Every Size (HAES), 28, 54, 80, 86, 105–7, 155, 169

health-care workers. *See* medical community
healthful eating: dieting *vs.*, 79–81, 185n10; Health at Every Size (HAES), 28, 54, 80, 86, 105–7, 155, 169; intuitive eating, 1, 65, 106
healthicization, 84–85, 86, 87
healthiness: as moral obligation, 39, 87–89
healthism, 87, 89
hegemonic masculinity, 80, 111–12, 115
Heron, Kristin E., 137
Hesse-Biber, Sharlene Nagy, 68, 71, 137
heterenormativity, 111–12
Heuer, Chelsea A., 41, 43, 165
Higgins, L.C., 65
high blood pressure, 1, 23, 80, 89, 103
hogging, 4–5, 114–15, 119, 173
homosexuality: identity and, 35; internalizing homophobia, 42; same-sex relationships, 125–26; visibility and, 11, 15
Hoppe, R., 85
Hot and Heavy: Fierce Fat Girls on Life, Love, and Fashion (Tovar), 27
Houy, Joshua, 171
Huff, Joyce, 14
humanist *vs.* feminist, 187n5
Huon, G., 65
Hurst, Shannon R., 123
hyper(in)visibility: about, 12–19; dating and, 134–35; diet culture and, 67–69; disease label of obesity and, 14–15; eating disorders and, 76; fatphobia and, 15, 38, 150–51; fear of fat and, 44–45, 55; healthcare system and, 86; invisibility and, 12; mind/body split and, 58; Othering

hyper(in)visibility (*continued*)
as, 12, 58; self identity and, 55; sensationalistic focus on health and, 47, 55; sexuality, 134–35; social surveillance and policing, 51–52, 62–64; in stigmatized groups, 161, 168–69; visibility spectrum, 166–69
hypersexuality, 28, 111, 112, 113, 133–34
hypertension, 21, 23, 56
hypothyroidism, 60, 91, 93, 163

identity. *See* self identity
individual responsibility, emphasis on, 3, 38, 39, 55, 82, 86–89, 117
industrialization and food, 39
inferiority, feelings of, 33, 38–39, 42–43, 46–48, 126–27, 158, 161–62
internalized oppression, 41–47, 54–55, 56, 57, 113–14, 117, 167–69
International Size Acceptance Association (ISAA), 26, 187–88n3
Internet trolls, 163
interviewees: Abigail, 146; Aisha, 90, 147; Alice, 64; Ann, 52, 105; Barbara, 78, 94, 98; Becky, 99–100; Beth, 73, 150, 153; Bonnie, 80–81, 121–24; Brenda, 125; Brooke, 38–39, 79–80, 98; Carol, 60–61, 70, 72–73, 107, 149; Carrie, 131; Cassie, 49–50, 50, 63, 117–18, 128, 143, 155; Cathy, 101, 103, 106; Claire, 63, 122; Claudialee, 83–84, 109; Dawn, 126; Elaine, 74–75, 76, 147; Elizabeth, 54, 116, 122, 145–46; Evelyn, 13–14; Fernanda, 42, 68–69, 91–93, 98–99; Jana, 133; Janet, 46, 62, 116, 144; Jasmine, 77–78; Jennifer, 1–2, 124; Jessica, 17, 42–43, 134; Karen, 42, 46, 148; Kathryn, 100–101, 129–30; Katrina, 71–72, 104, 129; Krista, 52–53, 103–4, 132; Linda, 37, 67–68; Lisa, 148, 149; Liz, 45–46, 51, 96; Lupe, 72; Mandy, 53–54, 65–66; Margo, 120–21; Marilyn, 39–40, 71–72; Marissa, 36, 48, 50, 64; Marsha, 80; Mary, 146; Meredith, 89–90, 115–16; Mindy, 132; Miranda, 62; Nancy, 77; Nicole, 50–51, 66, 74, 106, 118–19, 155; Paige, 93–94; Pam, 61, 96, 152; Patricia, 43, 44, 96–97; Rachel, 59–60; Rita, 101–2, 131, 144–45; Rochelle, 12, 40–41, 93; Sally, 90–91, 127–28; Sara, 46; Shannon, 123–24; Shawna, 51, 58–59, 98–99, 132; Sophia, 44, 105; Sue, 43–44, 104; Susan, 107; Tina, 48, 119, 129, 153; Tracey, 91, 105, 130; Veronica, 126–27; Wendy, 38, 74–75, 94–95
intuitive eating, 1, 65, 106
iron maiden torture device, 53
Izrael, Teshima Walker, 159–60, 170

Jennings, Laura, 9, 169
Jerant, Anthony, 22
Jersild, A., 33
Joanisse, L., 97
Joiner, Thomas E., Jr., 32
Jones, Substantia, 150–51
junk food, 22, 106–7, 155

Kalantar-Zadeh, K., 103
Katz, Sidney, 38, 138
Kent, Le'a, 19
Kiefer, Amy K., 123
Killer Fat (Boero), 4
Kim, Y., 138

kink community, 127–28
Kirkman, M. Sue, 22
Kitsuse, John I., 35, 36
Klein, D., 85
Koppelman, Susan, 119
Korenman, Sanders, 3, 171
Kristeva, Julia, 57
Kwan, Samantha, 14, 32, 87
Kyrölä, Katariina, 44–45, 183n1, 196

Lainscak, M., 103
Lamarche, B., 103
lap band surgery, 2, 39–40, 61, 76, 184n3
large, usage of word, 4
Latinas, 8–9, 32, 62, 91–93
laziness, stereotype of, 19–20, 31, 38–39, 44, 55–56, 66–67, 97, 134
LeBesco, Kathleen, 111, 151
Lepoff, Laurie Ann, 138
lesbians, 125–26, 168
less than, feelings of, 33, 38–39, 42–43, 46–48, 126–27, 158, 161–62
Levitt, Amanda, 163
Lewis, D. M., 137
Lim, J., 65
lipedema, 94–95, 163
Lipoedema: You Mean It's Not My Fault? (film), 95
looking-glass body, 15–16, 41
looking-glass self, 15–16, 41–42
Luedicke, Joerg, 20, 63
Lupton, Deborah, 88, 112
Lyons, Pat, 22, 88

MacGregor, M., 97
Maiman, L. A., 85
Malson, Helen, 87
Mancini, Henry, 151
marginalization. *See* discrimination; stigma and stigmatization
Marketdata Enterprises, 67
Maroney, D., 85

Martin, Michel, 159
masculinity: gender-roles norms and, 80, 111–12, 115, 132–33; humiliating women to achieve, 4–5, 114–15, 119, 173
Mason, Katherine, 171
Mayo Clinic, 91, 184n3, 184n6
McCarthy, Melissa, 170
McEvoy, Sharlene A., 171
Mead, George Herbert., 9, 33–34
media: beauty standards, 137; framing of obesity as disease, 2–3, 18–25, 43, 85, 111–14, 164–65; sexuality, 111–12; stereotypes reinforced by, 14, 20, 23–24, 51, 111, 170
medical community: antifat attitudes of, 1–4, 3–4, 61, 81, 88–89, 97–99, 140, 184n2; avoiding doctors and care, 22, 84–86, 88, 97–102; fixing bodies, focus on, 57, 59–61; focus on losing weight, 73, 76, 79; hyper(in)visibility fueled by, 14–15; on obesity, shifting views, 164–65; obesity viewed as epidemic by, 21–23, 85–86, 88–89, 97–99; physician-monitored diets, 73, 76; thinness, focus on, 39
medical equipment, 14, 49–51, 86, 99–102, 108–9
medicalization, 3–4, 84–85, 86, 99
Mellis, L. P., 85
mental illness, 84, 168; suicide, 39, 56, 163, 168
metabolism: caloric restriction and, 73–74; hyperthyroidism and, 91; weight cycling and, 80; weight gain in children and, 60
Meyerhoefer, C., 87
microaggressions, 49–50, 99
Mike & Molly (TV show), 170
Miller, Wayne C., 74
Millman, Marcia, 111, 187–88n4

Missing Bodies: The Politics of Visibility (Casper and Moore), 6–7
mistreatment and abuse: body shame and sexuality, 117–23; bullying and verbal abuse, 40–41, 43; feelings of deserving, 47, 48, 50, 55–56, 117–23, 134–35, 135; hogging, 4–5, 114–15, 119, 173; occurrence of, 24–25, 166–67, 184n8; in relationships, 4–5, 117–23; by sexual partners, 113–16. *See also* discrimination
Mitchell, Allyson, 151–52
mobility problems, 38, 59, 155
Moore, Lisa Jean, 6–7, 19, 165, 171
morality: health as moral obligation, 39, 87–89; judging others and, 50–51, 55
morbid obesity, 2, 102
mortality, 22
motorized scooters, 38
Muennig, Peter, 108
Murray, Samantha, 3–4, 31, 36, 60, 87, 88, 90, 94, 111, 154–56, 158, 159

National Association to Advance Fat Acceptance (NAAFA), 5, 25–26, 119–20, 139–41, 143–44, 153, 157–58, 174, 186n3
National Association to Aid Fat Americans, 139
National Institute of Health (NIH), 21
National Women's Studies Association (NWSA), 166
neoliberalism: cultural emphasis on health, 87, 89; health as a moral obligation, 39, 87–89; individual responsibility, emphasis on, 3, 38, 39, 55, 82, 86–89, 117
Neumark-Sztainer, D., 70

Newmahr, Staci, 128
"nocebo effect," 108
nonsexuality, 28, 111, 112, 117, 133–34, 170
"normalizing obesity," 164

Oakley, A., 180
obesity: childhood obesity, 41, 55, 57, 61–62, 83–84, 184n7; eating disorders and, 71–76; usage of word, 3
obesity, shifting views on: fatphobia and disease label, 162–65; medical views, 164–65; need for change, 161–62, 169–71
obesity as epidemic/disease: about, 19–25; AMA on, 83, 109; CDC on, 20, 21, 23–24, 87; criticism of disease label, 2–3, 14–15, 58, 83–86, 103, 183n4; discrimination fueled by, 24–25, 42–43, 55, 85, 112–14, 148–49, 159; epidemic, defined, 3–4; government focus on, 2–3, 20, 21, 87, 109; health care cost concerns, 87, 117; hyper(in)visibility fueled by, 14–15; media focus on, 2–3, 18–25, 43, 85, 111–14, 164–65; medicalization, 3–4, 84–85, 86, 88, 99; medical profession's focus on, 21–23, 85–86, 88–89, 97–99; political focus on, 2–3; poor health outcomes and, 21–22; sensationalistic framing of, 2–3, 18, 20, 103, 112–14, 164–65; "war on obesity," 4, 6, 20, 32, 42–43, 55, 169
Obesity Myth, The (Campos), 21
obesity paradox, 102–5, 108–9
objectification: losing weight and feelings of, 133; of men by society, 187n1; self-objectification, 58; visibility

and, 9; of women by men, 4, 113, 119–20, 125
ocular ethic, 7–8, 19, 166, 171
Oelbaum, Brenda, 152
Ogden, J., 85
Oldroyd, J., 22
Oliver, J. Eric, 21, 164, 165
online communities: antifat messages on, 163–64; fat activism via, 139–40; fat-o-sphere, 26, 139–40, 141, 143–44, 159
online dating, 121, 125
online reviewers, 163–64
open relationships, 127
Orbach, Susie, 113
Ortega, F. B., 22, 104
Othering, 10, 12, 17–18, 35, 39–40, 58, 166
Overeaters Anonymous (OA), 74
overeating: assumptions about, 19, 44; BED (binge eating disorder), 1, 63, 70, 71, 74–75, 78, 150; binge eating disorder (BED), 1, 63, 70, 71, 74–75, 78, 150; Binge Eating Disorder Association (BEDA), 101; caloric restriction and bingeing, 40, 73–74; secret eating, 74–75
overweight, usage of word, 3
Owen, Lesleigh, 49–50, 99

panopticon, 10
parents. *See* family
passing as thin, 35–36, 82, 143, 154, 183n3, 184n4
patriarchal values, 64, 79
Patsa, C., 103
Patton, G. C., 71
perceptions of others: looking-glass body, 15–16, 41; other's perceptions of fat and, 47–48, 50–51, 55, 123–26; self-identity and, 15–16, 41–42, 47–48, 55

Perez, Marisol, 32
persons of size, usage of word, 4
Peterson, Jaime Lee, 20, 63
pharmaceutical industry, 21
physician-monitored diets, 73, 76
physicians. *See* medical community
Pingitore, A., 103
Pitts, Victoria, 2, 79
Playing on the Edge: Sadomasochism, Risk, and Intimacy (Newmahr), 128
plus size, usage of word, 4
polyamory, 127
polycystic ovarian syndrome (PCOS), 40, 60, 93, 163, 184n6
Popular Culture Association (PCA), 166
Poretsky, Golda, 108
potlucks, 67–69
poverty: diabetes and, 21–23; weight gain and, 32, 40–41, 55. *See also* socioeconomic status
Powell, B., 3, 25
prednisone, 107
pregnancy, 4, 91–92, 94–95, 98–99
Preissler, Joanne, 5, 114
Pretty Porky and Pissed Off, 151–52, 159
Price, J. H., 85
Prohaska, Ariane, 5, 111, 113–15, 173
public health, 85, 87–88
public sex, 127
public spaces: college campuses, 45; eating in public, 58–59, 67–69; grocery stores, fatphobia in, 38, 58–59; restaurants, 49–50, 58–59; spatial discrimination in, 49–51
public transportation, 49
Puhl, Rebecca M., 15, 20, 31, 41, 43, 63, 83, 165, 171

race and ethnicity: African Americans, 32, 124, 159–62; cultural views on fatness, 32, 40–41, 55, 64, 154; diabetes and, 21–22; internalizing racism, 42; Latinas, 8–9, 32, 62, 91–93; sizism and racism, 42, 55; socioeconomic issues and, 32, 40–41, 55, 171–72; visibility status, 8–11; weight gain and, 40–41, 55
Rajaram, Prem Kumar, 11
Rand, C. S., 97
Read My Hips (Brittingham), 44–45
Reas, Deborah L., 75
Rebelos, E., 22
Register, C., 171
restaurants: eating in, 58–59; spatial discrimination in, 49–50
Rhode, Deborah L., 138
Riley, Kevin W., 88, 97
rodeo, 115
Rodin, J., 137
Rose, Nikolas S., 87
Rothblum, Esther, D., 3, 15, 24–25, 166
Roux-en-Y gastric bypass, 2, 76–77, 78, 89
Royce, Tracy, 117, 121

Saguy, Abigail C., 14–15, 19, 23, 24, 31–33, 33, 35, 42, 55, 71, 85, 88, 97, 113, 138, 140–43, 143, 150, 151, 163–65, 165
same-sex relationships, 125–26. *See also* homosexuality
Sanchez, Diana T., 123
Sartore, M., 171
Schallenkamp, Ken, 171
Schneider, Joseph W., 84
Schur, Edwin, 31
Schvey, Natasha A., 165, 171
Schwartz, Marlene B., 44, 97
secret eating, 74–75
Sedgwick, Eve Kosofsky, 31, 35, 142

self, defined, 33–34
self-acceptance: age and confidence, 132, 142; body/mind separation, 42, 52–58, 66–67, 129, 142; fat identity, embodiment of, 133, 141, 143–47, 149, 158–59; Health at Every Size (HAES) ideology, 28, 54, 80, 86, 105–7, 155, 169; identity and, 51–54
self-conception, 52–54, 55, 82
self-empowerment, 25–26; fat-o-sphere, 26, 141, 143–44, 159
self-esteem: age and confidence, 132, 142; appearance and, 8–12, 51–54, 55, 82; body/mind separation, 42, 52–58, 66–67, 129, 142; body shame and sexuality, 5, 117–23; effect of bullying on, 38–39; internalizing fat hatred, 41–47, 54–55, 56, 57, 117; less than, feelings of, 33, 38–39, 42–43, 46–48, 126–27, 158, 161–62; perceptions of others and, 15–16, 41–42, 47–48, 55
self-hatred, 39, 41–47, 42–43, 54–55, 142, 146, 167; internalizing fat hatred and, 41–47, 54–55, 56, 57, 117; overcoming, 133, 141, 143–47, 149, 158–59
self-identity: body as temporary, 34–37; body/mind separate from self, 42, 52–58, 66–67, 129, 142; coming out as fat, 35–37, 142–43, 154, 159; embodiment of fat, 133, 141, 149, 159; fat hatred, effects on, 31–35; fat identity embodiment of, 133, 141, 143–47, 149, 158–59; hiding self, 3–37, 82; identity defined, 33–34; internalizing fat hatred, 41–47, 54–55, 56, 57, 117;

looking-glass self, 15–16, 41–42; passing as thin, 35–36, 82, 143, 154, 183n3, 184n4; perceptions of others and, 15–16, 41–42, 47–48, 55; reflected acts and, 34, 47–48; self, defined, 33–34; self-acceptance and, 51–54; self-conception, 52; as subject and object, 9; visibility spectrum and, 8–12

Seo, Catherine, 95

Serpe, Richard T., 34

setpoint theory, 106

sexuality and sex: alternate sexual lifestyles, 126–28, 168; assumptions about fat women, 115–16, 126–27; BDSM (bondage, discipline, sadomasochism), 127; bisexuality, 126; body acceptance and sexual enjoyment, 126; body shame and, 5, 117–23; homosexuality, 125–26; hypersexuality, 28, 111, 112, 113, 133–34; literature on, 27, 186n10; nonsexuality, 28, 111, 112, 117, 133–34, 170

shame and guilt: body shame, 5, 41, 42, 117–23; public shaming, ineffectiveness of, 41

Silber, T. J., 32

Silberstein, L. R., 137

Sinding, C., 180

Sisyphus myth, 185n11

size acceptance movement: about, 25–27, 139; Adipositivity Project, 150–51; art as form of protest, 152–53; BBW (Big Beautiful Women) groups, 26, 146, 156; civil rights, 25, 140; coming out as fat, 35–37, 142–43, 154, 159; concerns about, 154–58; "doing fat" as activism, 150–53; fat activism *vs.* involvment in, 143–44, 147; fat identity embodiment of, 133, 141, 143–47, 149, 158–59; fat-o-sphere, 26, 141, 143–44, 159; Fat Underground (FU), 25–26; goals of, 140, 149, 159; Health at Every Size (HAES), 28, 54, 80, 86, 105–7, 155, 169; International Size Acceptance Association (ISAA), 26; membership in, 143–44, 147; National Association to Advance Fat Acceptance (NAAFA), 5, 25–26, 119–20, 139–41, 143–44, 153, 157–58, 174, 186n3; negative reactions to, 163–64; in online communities, 139–40; tensions within, 140–41, 157–58

size discrimination. *See* discrimination; fat hatred; fatphobia; mistreatment and abuse

sleeve gastrectomy, 76–77

Small, E. J., 103

Smith, Sally E., 157

social acknowledgment, 9–11, 141–42, 167

social capital, lack of, 15, 179–80

social markers, 8–9

social surveillance and policing, 10, 35–40, 51, 59, 62–64, 113

socioeconomic status: diabetes and, 21–22; poverty and weight gain, 32, 40–41, 55, 171–72; race and ethnicity, 32, 40–41, 55; thin privilege, 3, 10–11, 39–40, 59, 137–38; visibility spectrum and, 8–11; weight gain and, 32, 40–41, 55, 64–65

Solovay, Sandra, 166

Sorensen, T. I. A., 171

soul, cultural focus on, 52

spatial discrimination, 49–51

Squires, Sally, 21

Star, Susan Leigh, 18, 167
Steadham, Allen, 26
stereotypes: fat as lazy stereotype, 19–20, 31, 38–39, 44, 55–56, 66–67, 97, 134; fear of fat, 37–38, 44–45, 55, 57, 114–16, 117; harmful effects of, 161–62; media reinforcement of, 14, 20, 23–24, 46, 51, 111, 170; racial and ethnic assumptions, 8–9; racial and ethnic stereotypes, 32, 161–62; visibly seeing fat and, 31–32, 46, 60, 102. *See also* discrimination; "doing fat" concept
stigma and stigmatization: concepts of, 31; "covering" concept, 50; fat/bad and thin/good dichotomy, 112–13, 137–38, 157–58; medicalization and, 3–4, 84; obesity viewed as disease fueling, 2, 24–25, 42–43, 55, 58, 112–14, 148–49, 159, 183n4; Othering, 10, 12, 17–18, 35, 39–40, 58, 166
Stone, Gregory P., 9, 167
Storz, N., 65
Strauss, Anselm, 18, 167, 169, 178
stress, 56, 147, 171
Striegel-Moore, H., 137
stroke, 103
Strong4Life campaign, 41, 55, 184n7
Stryker, Sheldon, 34
study methods, 173–81; content overview, 27–29; motivation for, 4–6
study participants. *See* interviewees
Stunkard, Albert J., 74
Such a Pretty Face: Being Fat in America (Millman), 187–88n4
suicide, 39, 56, 163, 168
Sutin, Angelina R., 41, 165
Swami, Viren, 114
swingers, 127
symbolic interactionism, 15, 179

Synnott, A., 97

teachers, fatphobia among, 57, 59–60, 63
Teachman, B. A., 3, 24, 97
Tell Me More (radio show), 170
Terracciano, Antonio, 41, 165
thin, passing as, 35–36, 82, 143, 154, 183n3, 184n4
thinness: beauty and health equated with, 38–39, 53, 55–56, 63–64, 86, 150; beauty myth and, 53; mortality and, 22; need for shift in focus on, 169–71; passing as thin, 35–36, 82, 143, 154, 183n3, 184n4; sex appeal equated with, 111–12; sexuality and social norms, 111–15; visibility spectrum and, 8–12
thin privilege, 3, 10–11, 39–40, 59, 137–38
thunder, 145
Tischner, Irmgard, 10, 18–19, 58, 59, 87, 108, 166
Tovar, Virgie, 26–27
Tovèe, Martin J., 114
Trogdon, J. G., 87
Type 1 diabetes, 83–84
Type 2 diabetes, 21–22, 65–66, 83–84

Ulijaszek, Stanley J., 22
unmarked categories, 138
uterine cancer, 94

Vannini, Phillip, 15, 41
Veblen, Thorstein, 32
Ventura, E. Emily, 22
Very Low Calorie Diets (VLCD), 73
Victoza, 65–66
virginity, 53
visibility: disabled people and, 10, 11–12; fat pride and, 141–43; Othering, 10, 12, 17–18, 35, 39–40, 58, 166; social acknowledgment and, 9–11,

141–42, 167; as social control, 18–19
visibility spectrum: about, 8–12; emphasis on appearance and, 8–12; hyper(in)visibility and, 7–8, 12–19, 166–69; invisibility, 167–68; marginalized bodies and invisibility, 10, 11–12; materialization of bodies, 7; ocular ethic and, 7–8, 19, 166, 171; power and visibility, 9–10; thin privilege and social invisibility, 3, 10–11, 39–40, 59, 137–38
Vogelzang, N. J., 103

Wann, Marilyn, 3, 20, 26, 31, 84–85, 108, 143, 144, 151
Ward, Anna, 24, 31, 33, 35, 141–43, 150, 151
"war on obesity," 4, 6, 20, 32, 42–43, 55, 169
Waskul, Dennis D., 15, 41
weight and health: fat as unhealthy, 45–46, 89–95, 90–95; fat women's views on, 90–95; genetics and body size, 3, 21, 60, 149–50; healthy as moral obligation, 39, 87–89; relationship between, 19. See also obesity as epidemic/disease
weight-based victimization. See discrimination
weight cycling, 22, 65, 73–74, 80, 88–89, 179
weight discrimination, laws on, 170–71
weight loss: challenges to achieving, 3, 35, 79–80, 82; diet pills, 21, 65–66, 81–82, 85; eating disorders, 70–76; medical focus on, 73, 76, 79; motivations for, 1, 40, 45, 58, 69, 93, 96; regaining weight, 57, 65–67, 73–74. See also dieting; exercise
weight-loss surgery (WLS): about, 76–79; gastric banding (lap band surgery), 2, 39–40, 61, 76, 184n3; gastric bypass, 2, 76–77, 78, 89; lap band surgery, 2, 39–40, 61, 76, 184n3; pressure from family for, 63–64; pressure from medical profession for, 15, 85; risks and side effects of, 76–78, 85, 184n3; Roux-en Y gastric bypass, 2, 76–77, 78, 89; sleeve gastrectomy, 76–77
Weight of the Nation (TV documentary series), 19, 20, 22–23, 24
Weight Watchers, 63, 79
Weinstein, Rebecca Jane, 27, 186n1
West, Candace, 16–17, 47, 123
Wheeler, L., 138
Wiederman, Michael W., 123
Wiley, Mary Glenn, 34
Williams, D., 171
willpower. *See* discipline and control
Wolf, Naomi, 53, 64, 133
Wooley, S. C., 22, 88, 150
work-related diets, 68–69
World Health Organization (WHO), 83

Yanovski, S. Z., 75
Young, L. M., 3, 25

Zimmerman, Don H., 16–17, 47, 123
Zitzelsberger, Hilde, 11–12